T0385319

'A story of perseverance, the importance of advocating for yourself and how the kindness of strangers can have a huge impact. Having been aware of Tilly for a few years it's been fascinating to sit and read about her story in more depth. After years of not being listened to, I'm so glad Tilly is being heard now. A lesson to us all on what it is to have hope, even when we are at our most depleted. Shocking, brave and raw.'

— Giovanna Fletcher, author, podcaster, actress and activist

'Tilly writes beautifully, with such compassion. She has a wise understanding far beyond her years. The insight that she gives the reader is in depth and astonishing. It is delivered in such a relatable way and even with humour. A really important book for all of us.'

— Donna Ashworth, poet and author of *Wild Hope* and *Growing Brave*

'What a sensational read. A real, heartfelt and insightful look into the lived experience of someone managing their chronic health issues.'

— Dr Nighat Arif, GP, medical broadcaster and author of *The Knowledge*

'In becoming the expert that no one wants to be, Tilly Rose turns the worst prize in the raffle into the best, wittiest, most painful, most human quest to find the answer to a medical mystery that no one else can solve. This is a triumph of spirit over adversity. I found myself not only falling in love with its author but also rooting for her to find a cure. To have written it from the battlefield of illness is nothing short of a literary miracle. This book, like its author, is the dandelion that grows between the cracks. I loved it.'

– Abi Morgan (OBE), screenwriter, playwright
and author of *This is Not a Pity Memoir*

'I found this book both heartbreaking and uplifting all at once. A true story of resilience, hope and unwavering courage. A reminder to us all that life is worth living and that love really can conquer all.'

– Frankie Bridge, TV presenter and author of *Open*

'An inspiring account of a torturous patient journey. A recommended read for all.'

– Dr Ed Patrick, anaesthetist, comedian
and author of *Catch Your Breath*

BE
PATIENT

Life, loss and laughter from
behind the hospital curtain

TILLY ROSE

monoray

First published in Great Britain in 2025 by Monoray, an imprint of
Octopus Publishing Group Ltd
Carmelite House
50 Victoria Embankment
London EC4Y 0DZ
www.octopusbooks.co.uk

An Hachette UK Company
www.hachette.co.uk

The authorized representative in the EEA is Hachette Ireland, 8 Castlecourt Centre,
Dublin 15, D15 XTP3, Ireland (email: info@hbgi.ie)

Distributed in the US by Hachette Book Group
1290 Avenue of the Americas, 4th and 5th Floors
New York, NY 10104

Distributed in Canada by Canadian Manda Group
664 Annette St., Toronto, Ontario, Canada M6S 2C8

ISBN 978 1 78072 622 9

A CIP catalogue record for this book is available from the British Library.

Typeset in 12/19pt Sabon LT Pro by Jouve (UK), Milton Keynes.

Printed and bound in Great Britain.

3 5 7 9 10 8 6 4

This FSC® label means that materials used for the product have been responsibly sourced.

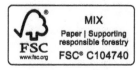

MIX
Paper | Supporting
responsible forestry
FSC
www.fsc.org
FSC® C104740

To Mum, for showing me night and day
that giving up is *never* an option.

CONTENTS

Part 3 – Chaos

PREFACE

Being ill is not a choice.

No one ever ponders their vision of the future and thinks, 'Hey, maybe one day I'll be a patient.' It's a raffle of the worst kind; the tragic tombola at the school summer fete that no one wants to enter and – having admired the prize selection (Sharon's curried apple sauce, Coral's handwoven placemats and Mitra's origami pets) – no one wants to win. In a cruel twist of fate, aged five, someone must have bought me one of those pink paper tickets and, as bad luck would have it, I won. I won a future of emergency admissions, endless waiting rooms, gruelling treatments and major operations. It really has turned into the prize that just keeps on giving.

Being a 'medical mystery' means I've now experienced every corner of the healthcare system for over 20 years. Along the way I've become highly qualified at two things: being *a patient* and being *very patient*.

When most people picture being in hospital, they think of needles, medication and procedures, but that's just surface-level stuff. At its core, being a patient is like being dropped headfirst into a social experiment you never signed up for. Growing up, you're constantly reminded not to talk to strangers; so why, the moment you're admitted to hospital, does it become acceptable to join them in a weird communal sleepover each night? You signed up for the treatment plan but no one mentioned the added extras. You may be in for 24 hours; you may be in for a month – but one thing I can guarantee is that you'll be exposed to life and human beings as you've never seen them before. This is a sleepover you'll never forget.

Be Patient is a story about becoming the expert no one wants to be. It is a tale about the rippling effect illness can have on those around you, as well as a broader comment on the fragility of humanity when faced with one of the most extreme settings in life. From monumental decisions to small acts of kindness, we will meet the people who shape the patient experience.

Now it's time to take you with me behind the hospital curtain. This should perhaps come with a warning sign: 'Be prepared to be unprepared'.

Here goes.

Part 1
MEDICAL MYSTERY

1

CLUES

'I'm going to need you to remove your knickers, my love,' Julie, the radiographer, says.

I was told I wouldn't have to move.

'Take as long as you need.' She smiles.

I contemplate how best to do this, settling on bending my knees and placing my feet flat on the mattress. I grip my thumb onto the elastic at the back of my leggings and tentatively begin to wriggle. My knickers make it halfway down my legs before it all feels too painful and I flop back onto the bed.

Out of the corner of my eye, I notice Julie lifting up a giant grey pole. I tilt my head to the side to get a better look. She squirts some clear jelly into her hand and begins rubbing the pole, in a sort of, well, *wanking* motion. What on earth is that for?

After taking a few deep breaths, I rather ingeniously hook my big toe around the edge of my pants and slide them off.

'This may be a little uncomfortable for a minute, sweetie,' Julie says, moving towards me.

In my pain-ridden state, I'm beyond caring. Within a few seconds, said pole is making its way between my legs.

'OK, the wand is now being inserted.'

It might sound like some New Age sex toy, but as the 'wand' enters my vagina it feels anything but magical. I'm now not only writhing in pain but writhing in pain with a giant pole shoved inside of me and three members of staff gathered around a screen analysing my organs. What is happening?

'So, can you point to the exact location of the pain?' Julie asks.

I try to gesture to my tummy and lower back.

'Sorry, can you just confirm exactly where the pain is?'

I'm now really struggling to move but flail my arms enough to point to my back, which is pulsating in sharp pangs.

'Loin,' I mutter. 'Doctor said loin pain.'

Julie stops circling the wand. The room falls silent. She traces her fingers over the request form. They all begin to talk in hushed whispers. The wand is swiftly removed. Julie passes me handfuls of blue paper towels to wipe away the excess lube dripping out of my vagina. There is now a pool of slimy gunk between my legs, sticking to my thighs.

'Tilly, my love, I'm afraid there's been a little mix-up.'

Turns out the doctor's handwriting was difficult to decipher. Turns out 'loin' and 'groin' look quite similar. Turns out I've just had a giant plastic pole inserted into my vagina for absolutely NO REASON.

'If it's any consolation, you have lots of eggs.'

The correct scan, on the correct body part, still fails to uncover the source of my agonising flank pain. Thankfully, it's decided that whatever is wrong is causing enough suffering to require super-strong painkillers and these transform me. By the next morning my body feels weak but I'm no longer in agony.

I've now survived night number one on the ward. It's always a relief when morning arrives. At 7am, the curtains are flung open and the light floods in. The ward is a hub of activity as nurses race around, the patter of their shoes sticking to the laminated beige floor. (Why *do* hospitals have beige floor? This seems like a total failing in the interior design. It pretty much guarantees a front-row viewing of the remnants of Edith's burst cannula and Marjorie's 'little accident' en route to the communal toilet.)

Nurse Safi bobs her head into my curtain.

'I heard about yesterday.' She laughs. 'If there was ever a case for the system to be digitalised . . . Then again, people pay good money for that in those swish private clinics! You got a free fertility service, Tilly.'

She's right. I should be grateful. Yesterday's unexpected vaginal ultrasound means I now know I'm the proud owner of an abundance of eggs. At 20 years old, my future is looking brighter than ever.

'I'm glad to see the pain meds have worked. You were in a real state last night.'

A stale, musty scent wafts down the corridor into our bay. This is quickly followed by a clatter of trolleys and the booming voices of the catering team, trying to tempt us with the various dishes on offer throughout the day. 'Fish and chips? Omelette? Chicken tikka masala?'

A man in a navy-blue polo-shirt hands me a flimsy paper menu. The options are quite literally endless. I can't take it all in. At 7am,

I don't know what I want for breakfast, let alone for lunch, dinner and pudding.

'Decided?' The man is now standing at the end of my bed, staring at me and impatiently tapping his foot. This is a highly pressured situation. There is no time to peruse. Without really looking I quickly tick a few boxes.

My roomies, on the other hand, are practically springing from their beds, salivating at the thought of putting their orders in. Patsy, in the next bed, phones her boyfriend, Ricardo, to inform him the food is 'damn good'.

'I think today I might give the allergen section a whirl,' I hear her say.

Last night, when it looked like she might be discharged, she went all out and ordered a 'supplementary snack' at 3am. At the very point the nurses are praying that patients stay asleep, the canteen is actively tempting us with cheese toasties. To be fair to Patsy, hospital changes your outlook; and you certainly can't accuse her of not seizing the moment. She is the ultimate '*Carpe Diem*' poster girl.

After breakfast comes the 'medication round', the inferior precursor to the real deal, the bit we're all waiting for, the 'ward round'. At this point, the whole atmosphere changes. Everyone begins talking in whispered voices, the previous frantic footsteps slow. It is clear that something big is happening.

A verbal, 'Knock, knock, knock,' and a light tap of my curtain indicate the doctors will now be paying me a visit. Chief Duck, aka the consultant, Dr East, approaches first. His ducklings shuffle behind. They line up in a semicircle around my bed, all eyes glued to me.

'How are you feeling today, Tilly?' Dr East asks, without looking up from his notes.

'Better than I was, thank you.'

'And why exactly are you here?'

'I became unwell again . . .'

'What does "becoming unwell *again*" look like?' He finally makes eye contact.

'Well, I have a bit of a complicated medical history . . .'

Dr East gestures for me to expand. I can now recite the spiel off by heart. I'm also expert enough to know that he has max five minutes to hear it, so I need to be as succinct as possible.

I rewind to age ten, the year my appendix burst and I could have died. The gunk all welled in my weirdly deep pelvis and I lived (a small victory). Then, I quickly jump to age sixteen when I had an 'emergency intestinal resection'. The surgeons cut my intestine in half, took a chunk out and sewed the two ends back together again. Then, just to really ensure that a hospital admission is never far away, recurrent pneumonias have been thrown into the mix, emphasis on *recurrent*. The worst bit: no one has any idea why the hell all this is happening to me.

I recount my story matter-of-factly. I've grown into this role over time and adapted to my 'new normal', but the truth is there's nothing 'normal' about it. This illness arrived without warning and now endlessly lingers, casting a dark shadow over the healthy, carefree ten-year-old who existed before. Had that girl known what she knows now, I'm not sure how she would have coped. Sometimes it's better not to know.

'Quite the medical mystery,' Dr East says.

I nod. Being a mystery in other walks of life is the pinnacle: that mysterious girl at school who lives on a canal boat and dyes her hair in accordance with the lunar calendar; that mysterious guy whose enigmatic texts make him irresistible; that mysterious colleague who claims to have spent her weekend doing laundry and watching TV with her cat, but turns up every Monday with a suspicious new love bite. These people are all mysterious in the way that they defy categorisation; you can't put them in a box or label them – and that makes them intriguing (and cool). Being a *medical* mystery is not cool. Mine is the bad kind of mystery, the one where everyone is trying to solve a horrific crime but the evidence has all been lost and the detectives are struggling to come up with new ideas. My case involves phrases like 'very unusual presentation', 'unexpected outcomes' and 'a confusing picture' – phrases no one wants to hear.

'And what would you *like* to be doing, if you weren't here?' Dr East asks.

At this point in the conversation, I know it's time to throw Oxford into the mix. I first visited the city on a day out with my parents when I was ten years old. We stumbled across a sign outside Balliol College, one of the University of Oxford's colleges, inviting the public to look around. Stepping into Balliol was like stepping back in time. As we walked through the quad, the sun pierced through the thick clouds and bounced off the chapel's stained-glass windows, forming a colourful rainbow across the trees. The greenest, neatest lawn I had ever seen was enclosed by tall stone walls dripping with ivy and framed with blossoming flowerbeds. Students wandered down the pathways, chatting to friends. I couldn't take my eyes off them. In that moment, I made up my mind that I was *going* to Oxford University.

That same year, I started to become unwell. I'd just moved to the local secondary school, but from day one I was hardly there. I'd sit in hospital waiting rooms rifling through cue cards. I'd lie in hospital beds reading set texts. I realised I could teach myself. It became the one thing I had control over and a distraction from the horrors of being so ill. 'Don't bother taking your GCSEs . . .' 'Don't put yourself under pressure . . .' 'I think university is a little unrealistic given your situation . . .' people said. They were right. It was a totally unrealistic goal, but I quietly held onto the tiny glimmer of hope that it wasn't impossible.

I proved everyone wrong. I got into Jesus College, Oxford to read English Literature and Language. At the point of meeting Dr East, I'm entering my second year. Doctors seem to like this; it shows I'm motivated, that I *want* to be well. A strange thing to have to prove and yet, 'Do you want to be in hospital?' is a question I've heard so many times that I now pre-empt it before it surfaces.

I *want* to be living that dream I've worked so hard for, delving into books on my incredible window seat overlooking the beautiful college quad and cycling around the city's charming stone walls. Instead, I'm the girl who stays up all night reading, knowing that the next day she could be in A&E. I'm the girl who owns a bright-pink bike who is never seen to ride it. I'm the girl who, on the outside, is 'always smiling' but who isn't always smiling inside.

'We're not sure what's causing the flank pain but our X-ray shows you do have another bout of pneumonia,' Dr East says.

The antibiotic tablets are no longer as effective as they once were. I'm now becoming more and more reliant on hospital I Vs.

'Why do I keep getting pneumonia?' I ask.

'We're not going to solve that here,' Dr East replies.

This is a response I'm now used to. Always worth an ask, though. One day, someone will have the answer.

'We'll treat the infection but much better to look into the cause as an outpatient.'

I know what Dr East is really saying is that he doesn't have the resources to try.

At midday, Nurse Safi shuffles towards my side table, holding the yellow A4 booklet containing my 'notes'. Given that my name is inscribed in bold black ink across the front and that the contents include every intimate detail about me, it would be reasonable for you to assume that I'd have at least a semblance of ownership over these but you would be wrong. Yesterday, they were accidentally left on my side table and when I dared to take a peek they were swiftly removed.

Safi hands me a little paper cup containing my lunchtime meds. It could be mistaken for a miniature shot but the contents don't glide down your throat like a tangy Apple Sourz. They get lodged and require several cups of lukewarm water from the blue-topped plastic jug to force them down. No one explains what they are, only that I *must* take them. Once Safi is satisfied that I've swallowed each pill, she moves onto my neighbour.

Chardonnay, the patient in the bed opposite, announces that she can't take tablets. She also has a lifelong fear of needles. Safi asks what she's eaten.

She can't eat. She's been vomiting.

The thing about being hospital neighbours is you really take the concept of nosy to a whole new level. I already have an in-depth knowledge of Chardonnay's daily routine: I know she calls her brother, Dean, at hourly intervals; I know she thinks Dr East is an 'arsehole' who isn't taking her seriously; I know she thinks it's a 'fucking joke' that her Hospedia – the TV, phone and entertainment centre above the bed – isn't working. I also categorically know that she has eaten. Last night, while I was attempting to get that rest everyone keeps telling me I need, she hosted a casual family reunion around the bed and ate two thirds of a bucket of KFC popcorn chicken, with a side of fries and Diet Pepsi, to be precise.

I'm just about to roll over and try to go back to sleep, when a healthcare assistant appears at the end of my bed.

'Would you like a wash?'

My blonde hair has already turned brown and is sticking to my head. There's no way I'm going to make it to the shower. I'm hooked up to so many machines I can't move.

She lifts up a scuffed blue bowl and crusty flannel.

'We call it a bed bath.'

'No thank you.'

'Is Bed 3 not washing?' an authoritative voice asks, from beyond my curtain.

'Wash REFUSED.'

Turning down the offer of a stranger giving me a 'bed bath'

has somehow translated into, 'This girl has a hygiene problem.' No doubt a new addition to my hospital notes.

A few hours later, Nurse Safi appears with a bag of IVs, which she hangs from a stand next to my bed.

'There you go, that will make you feel better.'

Within a few minutes, I get that familiar metallic taste in my mouth and know that they are beginning to flood my system. I'm aware that it will be only weeks, maybe even just days, before the pneumonia inevitably returns. This has become the cycle. The IVs aren't the cure; they just dampen it down for a while. Each time I come in, the doctors throw a few buckets of water over a roaring fire. Some of the flames turn to ash but the fire still burns. For tonight, though, the buckets of water are enough to make me smile.

I drift in and out of sleep as the antibiotics fill my veins. When I wake, Mum is sitting in the chair beside me. Dad and my boyfriend, Finn, stand behind her. I tilt my head up.

'You already look like a different person,' Mum says.

'That's our girl,' Dad nods.

Finn leans over and holds my hand (well, sort of – the cannula sticking out of my vein makes any romantic gesture a bit challenging). I gaze up at him, knowing I got all the luck that day we met in the first week of term. There's an Oxford tradition where, during week one, you get 'college married' to someone in your year. Then, the following year, when the next cohort of students arrive, each couple is allocated 'college children'. I spotted Finn in the King's Arms pub on our very first day. Our beautiful love affair progressed when, a few days later, he knocked on my door, got down on one knee and (college) proposed to me with a Haribo ring and a packet of heart-shaped Jammy Dodgers. Who said romance is dead? We later turned into a *real-life* couple. It would be a kind of fairytale, were it not for the ambulances, needles, blood and vomit rumbling away beneath the surface. To start with, I tried to hide this entire horror show from him, fearing that there would be no fairytale ending if he was faced with the reality of my situation, but as things have worsened that has become more and more difficult.

'I'm not going anywhere,' he says each time I question why he wants to stay with a girl who spends half her life in hospital.

He turns to me now.

'What are you going to do, Tills?'

Finn asks this every time I end up here.

'Beat it,' I whisper.

'More convincingly, please . . .'

'Beat it,' I say a bit louder.

He nods, satisfied.

'You're a legend, never forget that.'

Visiting hours are now coming to an end. I should be leaving with him. Instead, I'm stuck here. I feel an overwhelming wave of guilt. I can't be the girlfriend I want to be. I can't be the girl I want to be.

'I don't like leaving you,' Mum says.

'I'll be fine. I promise,' I try to assure her.

'Have you got your earplugs?'

'Yep.'

'Sleep mask?'

I dangle it in the air.

'OK, well I hope it's not too noisy.'

I laugh.

'It will be . . .'

She squeezes my shoulder. Dad leans over to kiss me on the forehead.

I wave goodbye to them all, then pop in my earplugs. I'm just about to pull my sleep mask over my face when I spot the sign above the sink.

Stay Safe. Wash your hands to stop the spread of germs.

I contemplate how washing my hands isn't going to keep me safe if Sheila in the bed opposite turns out to be a serial killer.

Lola, my night nurse, pokes her head through my curtain.

'Just wanted to check you're OK before I turn the lights out?'

'All good, thank you,' I smile. I mean, apart from the fact that the very circumstance of being in hospital means I'm now expected to roll over and go to sleep with a bunch of total strangers.

I notice Lola looks a little upset.

'Are *you* OK, Lola?'

She seems a bit taken aback but steps into my cubicle, drawing the curtain behind her.

'Not really.' A single tear drips down her cheek. She brushes her hand across it. 'One of my patients, Minnie, in the room next door. She just died.'

Not what any patient wants to hear. I prefer to focus on hospitals as a place people go to get better. I don't feel, in my present state, that I'm quite the right person to be counselling Lola, but it doesn't seem like she's getting much support elsewhere. She tells me how she tended to Minnie's every need, made her comfortable, spoke with her family, really got to know her. She even held her hand as she passed away.

At 8:47pm Minnie was pronounced dead. It's now 9:30pm and Lola is furiously attempting to wipe away her tears, hidden from view behind my curtain.

'It's all in the name,' she whispers. 'End-of-life care stops as soon as the life has ended.'

It occurs to me that if my auntie was at work and her colleague keeled over next to her, she'd be sent home immediately, given a few days' compassionate leave and probably be referred for counselling. The perks of finance.

Lola is a nurse. She signed up to work in the *caring* profession. She is contracted to care. To be good at her job, Lola must care *a lot*, but the contract stipulates that at 8:47pm Lola should have stopped caring. Dead bodies aren't a priority.

At 9:35pm, the ward sister calls through my curtain.

'Lola, where have you got to? Can you come and change Bed 2's catheter?'

It's true that not all superheroes wear capes, but I'm pretty sure that on occasion, even Batman was allowed to cry.

PATIENT SURVIVAL TIPS

- If a test or procedure feels a little odd (for example, pole up vagina), question it!
- The morning ward round is your one five-minute opportunity to ask the doctors any burning questions. Prep them in advance!
- In no other circumstance in life would you blindly take a pot of random pills from a stranger. Hospital is no exception. Ask what meds are in it.
- Having a distraction outside of patient life is essential.
- Staff also get sick, feel sad and have lives beyond the hospital wards. Never lose sight of that.

2

ZEBRA

Thankfully, I escape hospital just in time to celebrate my 21st birthday. On the night of my party, the lights go off and my relatives gather around. My auntie swans through the door, holding what at first glance, amid the candles and sparklers, appears to be a Victoria sponge. On further inspection, though, this is no ordinary offering. The lopsided cake is embellished with a mortifying montage of individual icing headshots of every single member of my family. Superimposed onto the centre of the shrine is a horrifically zoomed-in photo of 11-year-old me, my hair scraped back into a tight ponytail, two strands pulled in front of my face, held in position with some sort of gel product.

'Isn't your uncle clever?' Auntie gazes up at the mastermind behind the creation. Her very own Michelin-star chef.

'Look, there's Grandma Bridie.' She points. 'And there's your cousin Sophie.'

I burst out laughing.

'It's amazing,' I say. 'It really is.'

'A cake full of everyone who loves you,' Auntie smiles.

'Make a wish, Tilly.' Mum puts her arm around me.

I blow out the candles and close my eyes.

'What did you wish for?' Finn asks.

'I can't tell you or it won't come true.'

Mum looks at me, her eyes dewy. She knows what I wished for. It has been the same wish for the last 11 years.

I wish to get better.

All I want for my birthday is answers and all I get is more pills. Every day now I rattle through 30-plus tablets; there's barely room for food. Meds for pain, meds to stop me being sick, meds for skin reactions, meds to treat infections, meds to help me sleep, meds to control my heart, meds to support my lungs, meds to make my tummy work. Alongside this is the admin of patient life. It's starting to feel like the full-time job I never signed up for. With any other job, I could take a day off, plan in advance and mentally switch off, but being a patient isn't a role I can just leave behind. Some days it's more visible, other days it fades further into the background; but it's always there, tainting my every move.

It's the summer vacation and while my friends are off travelling the world, I'm travelling between medical appointments.

'It's beyond me . . .' 'I can't help you, I'm afraid . . .' 'If my clever colleagues haven't solved it, I don't think I'll be able to . . .'

Over the last 11 years, I've worked my way through virtually every department going: respiratory, gastroenterology, urology, endocrinology, gynaecology, radiology, cardiology, haematology, neurology. When they can't find the answer, the doctors pass me on. I'm sent from -ologist to -ologist like a hot potato.

'That's why you need a good GP,' our friends and relatives tell us.

There is a policy in England that anyone can register with a GP surgery. Whatever dire situation we may find ourselves in, GP surgeries are open to *everyone*. Well, almost everyone.

A week after my 21st birthday, a letter arrives in the post.

Dear Miss Rose,

I am writing to you, as the senior partner, on behalf of your General Practitioner.

We are saddened to see you have had so many health challenges over the last few years, resulting in multiple admissions to hospital. You have required numerous call-outs, particularly in recent months. Whilst we are committed to supporting our patients during these times, as I'm sure you will understand, we do have limited resources. We regret to inform you of our decision, that it would be better for all involved if you were to transfer to a new surgery which may be better able to manage your situation and provide continuity of care.

Kind regards,
Debra

Dear Debra,

Thank you very much for your recent correspondence.

This letter was, I must admit, a little unexpected. I wonder if you could perhaps give me any recommendations of local GP surgeries actively seeking ill patients?

Kind regards,
Tilly

Later that month, two more letters arrive in the post.

'You have got to be joking? I haven't visited them in 20 years,' Dad says, flapping one of them in his hand.

The GP has decided to fire not only me but my entire family.

Are you sexually active?
How many units of alcohol do you drink per week?
Do you take recreational drugs?

It seems my new GP is less interested in my medical history and more interested in how much of a legend I am.

I stare down at the sign-up form.

Help Us Get to Know You

I think of my body and then my illness. I prefer to view them as two entirely separate things. My body is the ship in the depths of the ocean, being brutally attacked by a raging storm. The sails have fallen, the ropes have torn, the deck is beginning to flood, but somehow the ship still floats. Everything is falling to pieces around me and yet I will not let it define me. I am the ship, not the storm. I am *not* my illness. Somewhere on that ship is the girl waiting for the lifeboat; but, for most people, she's too far from the shore to spot. They see only what is right in front of them. They see 'Tilly the patient' – and to be fair, when you 'get to know her' on this GP form, things don't look great. I have to tick 'Yes' to taking regular medication, I have to tick 'Yes' to having had major surgery, I have to tick 'Yes' to recent hospital admissions and I have to ignore the neat multiple-choice boxes in the 'Medical Conditions' section containing all the standard diagnoses. Instead, I have to ask for extra paper to write out a complicated sprawl of unanswered questions under 'Other'. You never want to be 'Other' in medicine.

In 1940, medical researcher Theodore Woodward coined the phrase, 'When you hear hoof beats, think of horses, not zebras.' The odds are that patients have common diagnoses rather than rare ones. On day one, I got Theodore Woodward's vibe; but 11 years down the line, he's totally screwed me over. I am now facing the hard truth that I am 100 per cent zebra. This comes with another hard truth: most medics prefer horses.

Thankfully my new GP, Dr Murphy, is different.

'Patients know their bodies better than anyone else,' he says in my first appointment. 'You've lived with this horrible illness for years now, Tilly, so how about you tell me what you think is going on here?'

So, I tell him. I tell him that I was perfectly well, before being struck down with appendicitis and then my first pneumonia aged ten. I tell him that this is a physical illness that in some way responds to antibiotics. I tell him that logic tells me there must be a reason why I suddenly needed an emergency bowel resection (not exactly normal). I tell him that 11 years on, I am finding it hard to hear the words, 'It won't be that; it's very rare.' Words that mean zebras face extinction where horses do not.

'If it wasn't rare, wouldn't we have found it already?' I pose to Dr Murphy.

He nods.

'I think you're right, Tilly. Now, I don't profess to have the answer but I can assure you, I will try my best to get these clever consultants to find it.'

Will he try, though? Will he really try?

When this illness first started, I entered each medical appointment full of hope. *This doctor could be the one, the one to solve the puzzle.* I'd pin everything on those meetings, nervously sitting in the waiting room, quietly asking the universe for this to be the day it all changed. Now, 11 years on, nothing has changed. I have learned the equation. Hope gets you through but unfulfilled hope leads to despair. Hope is a comfort but it also leaves you exposed. If you have no expectation, you can't be disappointed. Lately, I have been scared to hope.

'I'll make a few outpatient referrals for you,' Dr Murphy says.

I think of something Mum has so often said to me: 'It only takes one person. Only one person needs to care, Tilly.'

I look at Dr Murphy. He has kind eyes. I take a deep breath and today I choose to hope again.

*

A few weeks later, I'm sitting at my desk at uni when a letter arrives informing me about a new gastro appointment. Dr Murphy has stuck to his word and referred me on for more investigations. I'm unbelievably grateful but the letter is an intrusive reminder that, even when I'm not actually lying in a hospital bed, my illness is constantly there, threatening to disrupt my life.

From day one at university, I so desperately wanted to be known as 'Tilly', not 'Tilly the patient'. Over the years, this has involved becoming an expert juggler. It has been impossible to hide my hospital stints but no one really knows the extent of what's going on; the meds, the appointments, the equipment. Mum creeps through the quad in the dead of night to deliver my prescriptions, avoiding any prying eyes. Where most students' cupboards are stuffed full of books, stationery and clothes, mine are bursting with medical equipment, pills and emergency protocols. I spend my life being ahead of the game, getting the work done immediately in case there is another disaster around the corner. I always have a list of excuses at my fingertips – 'Oh, sorry, I already have plans tonight . . .' – when really I'm rather tragically stuck in my room. No one knows I spend my evenings lying on my bed with a nebuliser (inhalation machine) strapped to my head to ease my gunky lungs. No one knows I sleep with my feet up in the air on five pillows, to stop the blood pooling in them at night. No one knows that if I were to climb the stairs every day, the pneumonias would spiral out of control. No one knows how bad things are getting.

Finn knows more than the rest but even he doesn't see it all. I'm scared that if anyone really knows the truth, the façade will crumble and then I will crumble. Juggling is exhausting but this double life allows me a semblance of normality and I need to hold onto that to get through.

Today, as I attempt to scurry across the quad, I bump into my friend Pia. We're both reading English and bonded in our first-ever class, when it became apparent that all the other students had a grasp of Latin tenses and we had none. This threw us both into full-on panic mode. We were certain Oxford had made some sort of mistake in choosing us and it was only a matter of time before they realised. So, we headed back to my room, put on the kettle, curled up in my bed and commiserated over many a cup of tea. From that moment on, we became inseparable, which makes trying to hide this whole hospital life even trickier.

'Where are you off to?' she asks.

'Heading to the library,' I lie.

'OK. Will you be at dinner?'

Good question. That all depends how many patients are in the waiting room.

'Planning to be,' I smile.

I wave goodbye and then pause for a moment, waiting for her to turn the corner. I wish I was heading to the library. Instead, Mum is down the road, ready to drive me to my gastro appointment. This will be my fourth appointment of the week. This illness is now robbing me of so much time. My days are fractious; I end up trying to plan essays in the car and wade through reading lists in waiting rooms. My mind is constantly hopping. By the time I arrive back at university after each appointment, I've generally fitted in a whole day elsewhere. I'll have planned beforehand, travelled to the hospital, sat in the waiting room, navigated the appointment, potentially had some tests, waited at pharmacy to collect prescriptions, discussed the appointment with Mum afterwards and, finally, travelled back. Meanwhile, my friends will have simply spent the afternoon in the library. I feel like I'm cramming in a second life alongside my degree.

'It's not fair,' Mum says, leaning over to give me a hug as I sit down next to her ready for the 30-mile drive to a hospital we've never been to before.

I shake my head.

'You should be out there with all of them.' She points across the street.

It's a bright and sunny November morning. I gaze up at the city's 'dreaming spires' rising like a melody against the milky-blue sky. The street is bustling with students, some dawdling, others running, the cold air spiralling in a white mist in front of their faces. Tinny bells ring out as bikes swerve around the corners. The scene has an almost electric energy, so incongruent with where I'm headed.

'I don't want to go,' I whisper. Even as I say it, I know I will go. I'll go as many times as I need to, in order to get my life back.

'I know it's horrible, Tilly, but this could help them sort you.'

I frown and pull an annoyed face. Mum is the one person trying to help me, the only person really trying to crack this. More and more of her life is becoming devoted to days and nights spent online, researching my weird array of symptoms; and yet, in this moment she is the person that I'm annoyed with. The truth is there is no one to be annoyed with. That's part of the problem. I want someone to blame.

I make a grumbling noise that translates to, 'I hate that you are right,' then look up at her and flicker a smile – a smile that says, 'I love you.' Deep down we both know that I'll do anything to feel better. Mum leans over and squeezes my shoulder, before turning the ignition and beginning our fourth road trip of the week.

On arrival at the hospital, we circle the ugly grey building in the centre again and again. It quickly becomes clear that we are lost. By the cars filling the road and the people gathering at the various side doors, it seems we are not alone. The 'Welcome' sign is misleading. No one can work out how to get in. We find ourselves at a complete standstill in a traffic jam. Traffic jams are always annoying but this traffic jam happens to be blocking the entrance to A&E, so in addition is a sort of life/death barrier. Eventually, the driver in front has had enough. She pulls up onto the kerb and dumps her car on the grass verge. It turns out survival chances are greater if you walk to A&E.

We finally make it into the hospital and begin following the signs to gastroenterology – that is, until they disappear.

I collar a lady in blue scrubs walking towards us.

'So sorry, we're looking for the gastro clinic – would you know where that is?'

'If I had a penny for every time I was asked that in this corridor . . . It was decorated last year,' she adds, as if that somehow explains it.

I'm not sure what she's getting at.

'They forgot to put the signs back up.'

She kindly gestures for us to turn right, walk down another long corridor, take two floors up in the lift, walk across the bridge, ignore the second door on the left – which says 'gastroenterology' but is, naturally, orthopaedics – then walk through a set of heavy double doors.

'There should be a reception desk right in front of you.'

'Thank you so much, you're a real lifesaver,' I smile. Only now do I notice her badge. Turns out she *is* a lifesaver. Well, she would be. Instead, this surgeon is having to moonlight as a hospital satnav.

We arrive with just minutes to spare. A plastic whiteboard, etched with messy marker ink, reveals there are four doctors holding clinics today. I look around the room at my competitors. Ultimately, we all know that everyone wants to see Dr Shafiula, the consultant.

'Tilly Rose.' I hear my name being called.

I'm allocated 'one of his team'.

Dr Aran begins by enquiring about my medical history, then tries to get a bit of a sense of 'me', asking whether I'm working or studying, before moving onto my symptoms. I'm now pretty familiar with this drill and always prepare for the appointments in the same way. I write out brief bullet points on my medical history and a concise list of symptoms and questions. I know appointments are short and how important it is to use time as efficiently as possible. There's always so much information, it's impossible to remember everything that's said, so Mum and I always come armed with a notepad and pen to record any ideas or follow-up tests that are mentioned. That way we have a record to look back on afterwards.

'Now, today I want to have a little chat about your diet,' Dr Aran begins.

I smile at Mum. I've pre-empted this and already put together a list of all the diets I've tried. Over the last few years, we've delved into the 'free-from' life with vigour: sugar-free, dairy-free, gluten-free, lactose-free, high fibre, low fibre, low sodium. We are now converts to smoothie life too; from superfood berries to spinach and asparagus cleanses, dashes of chia seeds and sprinkles of turmeric, we've done it all. Though I did have to put my foot down when I found Mum peeling cloves of garlic. Some things should not be juiced.

Along the way, we have learned some key life lessons: everything tastes better with sugar (a sad truth); 'rice cakes' should be taken to court over false advertising (they in no way resemble cakes); and the 'simple smoothie bowls' in social-media photos are never simple (cue a trip to an independent wholefoods store to buy vanilla protein powder, cacao – not cocoa – nibs, arrowroot flour, steel-cut oats, fresh pesticide-free fruit and coconut water. Yes, you even have to buy the water).

'Well, I know many patients think just a few cokes, chocolate bars and packets of crisps here and there won't do any harm, but we can end up consuming a lot more than we think.'

'I don't eat any of that,' I say.

I lift up my top to reveal my ginormous tummy ballooning against my skinny frame.

'What is it?' I ask.

I'd say I look about six months pregnant. If I put on a maternity dress and cupped my hand over it, I think I could persuade everyone to host me a baby shower.

'We're not entirely sure what's going on here but we think that, ultimately, it's best that you stop eating,' Dr Aran says.

Have I heard him right? Dr Aran has presented this with the casualness of just asking me to cut back on a little chocolate.

'No food at all?'

Feels like a bit of a leap. If your legs hurt, would the doctors say, 'We'd suggest you just stop using them – please sit down from now on'?

'Don't worry, this liquid nutrition is just as good as food.'

He pulls out a white bottle, patterned with a garish purple design. Scrawled across the front is the line 'For Medical Purposes Only'. He notes my expression.

'Just as good . . . *in a nutritional sense.*'

He lifts up the bottle.

'They do come in ten flavours. So, you could have vanilla for breakfast, strawberry for lunch and forest fruits for dinner.' He pauses. 'Hey, you could even add in a chocolate for pudding, Tilly.'

PATIENT SURVIVAL TIPS

- Never stop wishing when you blow out the candles on your birthday cake. Hope will get you through.
- Don't underestimate the power of a good GP. They can be your best ally when things go wrong.
- Hospital car parks are a maze. Clinics often won't just 'squeeze you in' if you're late, even if it is because their car park is a joke. Be on time.
- Write lists before appointments. This is your one chance to ask those all-important questions.
- You may be a zebra but remember 'rare' does not mean *impossible.*

3

BATTLE

Over the years, my juggling act becomes even more impressive; more and more balls are thrown into the mix and yet somehow, with the help of my expert sidekick (aka Mum), I manage to keep them all up in the air. My performance gets slicker. I perfect a schedule that works for me; well, for my body anyway. This involves sleeping in every morning until at least 11am. Two years on and the college breakfast buffet is still a complete mystery to me. Mum continues to covertly fill my fridge with vitamin shots and supplements. I hold my nose and ritualistically knock these back between meals. Then there's exercise. Medical science says it helps pretty much every condition going but my body calls bullshit. Over the years, I've worked out a pattern: the more I move, the more I get pneumonia. I'm not talking going on a run or rowing a boat; I'm talking climbing the stairs or walking to the library. I can do it in the moment but a few days later, that dry cough emerges – the dry cough that leads to the chesty cough and then, generally, to a two-week stint in hospital. I don't get strong and toned, I get weak and ill. It's just not worth it.

I try to stay as still as possible. While other students enjoy the magic of the Oxford libraries, I quite literally roll from my bed to my desk, assuring my friends that I'm simply more productive in my room. My relationship with Finn pretty much revolves entirely around these four walls. Everyone does their own thing in the day and the Oxford expectation that we're glued to our desks means I hardly appear any different. No one really goes out for dinners or heads out on dates. We are like all the other couples; we chill in my room, watch TV and swing by hall, a few metres from my room, for food. Plus, given its prime location (and the constant supply of chocolate biscuits delivered by Dad), my room becomes the resident tea spot. This proves ideal for me. I can stay still as a statue and my friends all pop by.

Despite all of this, I still spend far more time agonising over my social calendar than I do any of my essays. Essays I can do from my desk, but nights out are trickier. I have to walk to the club, dance among the sweaty bodies, finish with the group trip for that essential post-night-out kebab and then miss out on vital sleep time. It becomes a constant toss-up. Is this night out worth ending up in hospital? Is this party worthy of a pneumonia? More often than not, my answer is *yes*. My refusal to give in means the juggling balls are getting heavier. After rounds and rounds of even more tests, the medics still have no idea what's wrong with me. The IV antibiotics are becoming less effective. The liquid diet has done nothing to stop my growing tummy. By the time I enter my final year at uni, it's all beginning to feel futile.

*

'Tilly's just through here,' Mum says to the two paramedics entering my room.

I'm both relieved and mortified. *Everyone* will have seen them.

Finn stands in the corner of my room looking shell-shocked. Whereas Mum has had years of experience dealing with ambulances, this is his first. His face is pale. He looks like he might faint. He'll be needing the stretcher next to me, the way things are going.

I'm now in a foetal position on the bathroom floor. It's weird, isn't it, how whatever age you are, everyone reverts to being a baby when afflicted with pain?

'How bad is the pain on a scale of one to ten?' the male paramedic asks.

I'm crying and being asked to determine whether these are 'pain-level five tears' or 'pain-level nine tears'. It suddenly feels weak to say ten. What do the numbers even mean? I wonder where a stubbed toe would sit. Excruciating for a second, like literally enough to take your breath away, but no one ever got prescribed morphine for a stubbed toe.

'Seven,' I murmur between rapid gasps of breath. My chest pain is enough to make it hard to speak. Seven seems reasonable.

'Right, let's get a drip up,' the paramedic says.

I've hit the jackpot. Seven has them whizzing me straight out to the ambulance. I feel bad for those patients who soldier on with 'pain-level six' and are, presumably, left writhing at home.

The downside is that there is only one route out to actually *reach* the ambulance. We exit through the quad, which is basically a goldfish bowl. It could not have more windows if it tried. All eyes will be on me.

'It's OK, Tilly,' Mum whispers. She knows this is my worst nightmare.

'Oh, wow, was your room home to Harold Wilson?' the male paramedic asks, noting the plaque on my door.

I attempt a nod but the effort of lifting my head is too much.

While Harold no doubt meandered across the quad in heated political debates, prepping for his role as future prime minister, I'm being pushed out of the same room in a rickety wheelchair with a cardboard sick bowl on my lap.

I begin to shiver. The female paramedic drapes a thin blue blanket around me. This excuse for a blanket has more holes than actual material. I pull at a piece of loose thread and twist it around my finger. Mum and Finn walk by my side. I don't look up. We finally reach the ambulance, parked up on the bustling Turl Street. All the pedestrians slow as they approach. It's like when there's a car crash, followed by a huge traffic jam. When you reach the scene, it usually turns out the crash was cleared hours ago. The backlog is, instead, caused by our strange human fascination with catastrophe. Everyone stops to have a good look before getting on with their day. I am now the car crash.

'Only one of you can join us,' the male paramedic says.

I point to Mum. I need my mum right now.

Finn squeezes my hand. 'I'll be there as soon as I can.'

I'm placed onto a hard, plastic stretcher. A series of seatbelts are strapped over my body, caging me in.

'Move, mate, move,' the paramedic shouts from the front of the ambulance, as we head off.

Please move, please. The ambulance rumbles and each bump

has me squealing out. Every few minutes my body automatically flings forward to cough and bring up mouthfuls of acidic saliva. I'm desperate to reach the hospital.

'You OK?' The female paramedic in the back leans forward and clasps my shoulder.

I'm so far from OK.

She keeps assuring me that 'we're nearly there' but there are no windows, so I don't know whether to trust her. Eventually the ambulance slows.

'We're here now, Tilly.' Mum holds my hand.

The back doors open and a wave of cold air engulfs me. My teeth chatter together. I'm wheeled down a ramp onto the concrete car park. The stretcher vibrates across the bumpy surface. We enter a stark corridor and stop in front of a pair of heavy double doors. The paramedic does a quick handover to the nurse.

'Tilly Rose, 21 years old, medical history of repeated pneumonias and bowel surgery. Chest pain, cough and heart rate up at 130. Mum says this is pretty typical. It's likely she'll need IV antibiotics. We've administered anti-sickness and fluids.'

The nurse nods and takes the piece of paper containing my notes.

'Really hope you feel better soon, sweetheart.' The paramedic leans over my shivering body. 'Before we go, would you mind if we just borrowed that blanket back?'

A&E waiting rooms are always full to bursting. Everyone wants in, but there isn't enough space for everyone. This club has to get more exclusive. Enter *triage*.

Triage is a bit like taking an exam to determine whether you are ill enough to get through to the next round. The triage nurses effectively play a 24-hour round of true or false. If there's at least a 60 per cent chance you're telling the truth, you'll most likely pass. The really high achievers will be allocated a bed. Those who just scrape through will be lucky to get a chair in the corridor.

The only way to jump the queue is to rock up in an ambulance. This makes you hospital royalty, the ultimate VIP. Well, that's the idea anyway.

'You're not going anywhere,' the nurse says to my paramedic. 'Until she's actually admitted to resus, she remains under *your* care.'

Today, it turns out, the hype has got out of control. There are queues not only for triage and A&E but also for resus – where patients with life-threatening conditions are taken. Far from being granted speedy access, the ambulance VIPs are now directed to a separate queue down a narrow corridor.

'Join the back please,' a nurse says.

This involves a tricky manoeuvre of my bed to *number eight* in the queue. My head is now resting against a toilet door.

'This is madness,' Mum says. We've queued in A&E waiting rooms before but an ambulance-bed queue is a new low. Paramedics are now lining the corridor. 'Are you not allowed to leave?' Mum turns to them.

'No, our shift finished half an hour ago but we'll be here until we can officially hand Tilly over.'

Instead of switching on their blue lights and racing off to emergencies or heading home after their shift, paramedics up and down the country are now being forced to spend their nights and days manning hospital corridors.

'It's bonkers,' the male paramedic says. 'And where are the obs machines? We can't have a scenario where we can't monitor patients in the resus queue.'

'Well, that *is* the scenario,' the nurse responds. 'There aren't enough machines.'

Eventually, the female paramedic sources one. She leans over to wrap the cuff around my arm. I glance at the machine. It's covered in red liquid. It's covered in blood. Someone *else*'s blood. There's a little paper sticker hanging off it. I note the date. Last cleaned, last year. I'm too ill to really care.

'How long do you think Tilly might be here?' Mum asks.

My body is hanging limply over the cardboard sick bowl. I'm repeatedly retching. My hair is wet through. I just want them to do anything they can to make it all go away. I want it all to stop.

'Sometimes it's up to an hour.'

'I've texted Dad and Finn, Tilly. They are on their way.'

'They won't be allowed in here,' a nurse interrupts. 'And you'll have to go now, Mum. We can't have visitors blocking the corridors.'

'Oh, I can't leave you here, Tilly.'

'I'll be OK, Mum,' I whisper. She leans over and strokes my head. 'Honestly, you go,' I say. 'Escape this place.' I attempt a smile, glancing around at the grim hospital corridor.

'There's nowhere else I would rather be, Tilly.'

She says that a lot, my mum. 'There's nowhere else I would rather be,' is a line I have heard her utter in dungeon A&Es, on open wards for weeks on end sleeping in a chair, in waiting rooms and ambulances. On the days when it all feels too much and I crumble under the weight of it, she tells me that she is exactly where she needs to be, right beside me.

The nurse is now hovering by my bed, waiting for Mum to leave.

'Keep your phone by you,' Mum says. She delves into my hospital bag and pulls out my charger, placing it on the blanket next to me. 'I love you, little one.' However old I am, I will always be her 'little one'.

Before she goes, Mum hands me my little pink quartz stone. She gave it to me as a good-luck charm when I first ended up in hospital all those years ago. After she leaves, I lie alone for hours in the cold corridor and hold that little stone like my life depends on it. In front of me lies a lady in around her sixties I'd say. Her daughter stands beside her, holding her hand. To start with I wonder why she's been allowed to stay. Then I overhear a conversation that makes it all too clear. The lady lies silently in the middle of the mayhem. There is no screen, no curtain surrounding her. A doctor appears and kneels on the floor next to her. It's impossible not to hear his words. He is telling her she will soon die. He is discussing palliative care in a public corridor. A queue of beds and trolleys overlook her; patients manoeuvre past her with drips while paramedics, nurses and healthcare assistants frantically dart between us all. I don't want to see it. I don't want to think about it. I want to block it all out but there is no escape. Wards and corridors don't come with neat little age bands like 'PG', '15' and '18'; each time you come in, you have no control over which story is going to unfold.

I turn to face the wall and feel the tears begin to rise in my throat.

There is no ideal way for this scenario to play out but I can't imagine this is how the doctor, the daughter or the patient want it to be.

Please, please send all the positive energies to that lady, I whisper to my little quartz stone. I am perhaps voicing my own fears, as much as hers. She represents my greatest fear of all: the moment the medics say there are no more options left. A moment I dread, a moment that no longer feels like a distant nightmare but a very real possibility.

I rub my little stone between my thumb and forefinger. I quietly assure the universe that I'll give back, I'll make sure my life means something. I bargain with it, as if by being a better person I'll somehow change my fate. I'm not sure it really works like that, though. I've seen so many good, kind people struck down with awful situations. I've seen others who appear to have it all moan about their seemingly perfect lives. So maybe it's all just random, unpredictable chaos.

I'll think about my stone later. I'll think about how it can't have really been listening. I'll think about how it let me down.

By the time I make it into A&E, precious time has been wasted and my body is now beginning to spiral out of control. It's as though someone has pressed a button and it has suddenly realised it is really, really ill. So ill, in fact, that my veins have disappeared. I've become very dehydrated, making my veins difficult to uncover. Equally, they are pretty fed up with being repeatedly battered and keep collapsing from overuse.

'We need to get blood out of her,' the doctor says.

Everyone knows my veins are in there somewhere, but they are playing a crafty game of hide and seek. This game requires the full concentration of everyone involved. I'm still shivering from hours spent in the freezing cold corridor. The nurses start filling plastic gloves with hot water. They balance these makeshift hot-water bottles up my arms in an attempt to dupe my veins into emerging. My veins are having none of it. After seven failed needles into my hands and arms, they resort to my feet.

'This will hurt, love, but it will make you feel better.'

The nurse pierces my foot. The vein instantly collapses. Within a few seconds the needle is back out.

'We're going to have to call Mike.'

In between another round of vomiting, I look up and there he is.

'Mike is an *army doctor*.' The nurse smiles.

I think this is supposed to be a comfort, but it concerns me a little that my body is now considered enough of a war zone to bring in the *army*.

Mike approaches Bay 3 and asks everyone else to step aside. I am now shaking uncontrollably.

'Tilly, Tilly, look at me please.' His voice has a soothing quality but also an assertiveness that refuses to be ignored.

I force my head up. Dangling in front of me is his RAF lanyard. Mike holds my face in his hands and talks me through the plan. Mike and I are comrades. We are about to head into battle together. He wants to ensure that we are on the same page.

'What we're going to do next isn't going to be nice, Tilly. I need you to promise me that you'll stay really still. Can you do that, Tilly?'

I nod.

'Nurse Vardaizo is going to hold your hand. I want you to keep looking at her.'

I nod again.

Mike is totally in control and that is exactly what I need.

'You must not move, Tilly.'

I clench my jaw, tighten my fists and fix my eyes on Nurse Vardaizo. The weapon is deployed. I let out a terrorising scream.

'Victory,' he cheers.

Mike – my hero, my commander – has invaded a territory no one has been brave enough to tackle with a needle before. I look down at the scene of battle.

Mike has conquered my groin.

I lie very still on the bed and glance down at my body, now littered with balls of cotton wool stuck down with jagged strips of masking tape. A dull ache radiates from my groin. The freshest needle mark across my foot seeps blood. The older pricks across my arms are already beginning to bruise. I know that by tomorrow my skin will be a mottled purple mesh. By next week, these will have turned into deep opaque stains. To the outside world, they will look worse; but they won't hurt so much by then. Around each bruise will be a sticky line of glue, clinging on long after the masking tape is removed. The glue will turn grey, permeated by the grease and sweat and dirt from the hospital – a sign that I am too ill to wash. When I do finally shower, the glue will put up a fight. I'll attempt to rub it away, leaving my skin red raw. I'll dig my nails into it to try to scratch it off.

When friends and family see me, it will be my bruises that will stop them in their tracks; a visible sign that I have been through a battle: these are my wounds. For once, my illness won't be invisible. I have learned that humans often have to see something in order to feel it. And yet, what they cannot see is that it is the bruises on the inside that hurt the most. I hold my pink quartz stone in my hand and think of the lady in the corridor. I wonder where she is now.

In the aftermath of battle, it is hard to feel human. I am like a slab of meat in a butcher's shop.

Mum, Dad and Finn have now been allowed in and are all gathered around my bed.

'I wish I could take it all away, Tilly.' Mum strokes my cheek.

Dad looks across at me, helpless tears in his eyes.

'My brave little soldier,' he says.

He is right. I am a soldier. I seem to be fighting a futile battle, full of uncertainty. Yet, when I look across at them, there is one thing I am certain of.

I am loved.

PATIENT SURVIVAL TIPS

- Patient life can turn into a life of pretending. 'It's OK that I can't eat . . .' 'It's OK that I've missed weeks off uni in hospital . . .' 'It's OK that I've spent half my day at a medical appointment . . .' It's really not OK and it's OK to say that.
- Your phone is no good if you don't have a charger.

- Olive oil + a piece of cotton wool = the ultimate hack for removing the sticky plaster glue.
- At times, your heart may hurt but your compassion will grow.
- It's hard to imagine that you will smile or laugh again after a battle. Believe that it will happen.

4

'ARE YOU BETTER NOW?'

F ollowing Military Mike's heroic intervention, two bags of IV antibiotics are swiftly administered and, as always, begin to work their magic. The doctor on duty in A&E swings by my bedside to break the news that I will now be heading to Ward 9C.

'We're going to have to pop you in a side room to start with, just until we confirm you're not infectious.'

He presents this hesitantly, as if I might be in some way disappointed. I guess for most patients being 'infectious' isn't exactly goals. Little does he know, I want to spring from the bed, wrap my arms around him and kiss him. I don't because one, that would be weird and two, I know from previous experience that it's best to keep my head down at any mention of a 'side room'. I've *never* been infectious in the past, but I'm not about to share this information and risk destroying this golden opportunity to get a proper night's sleep. I know only too well that I probably have only 24 hours of 5-star luxury before being moved to the open ward (aka communal sleepover from hell).

Three days later, I am, somehow, still living the side-room dream. There are no signs that I'm infectious, so I like to think my good fortune is because I've played the role of the perfect patient (in other words, I've kept quiet, been totally undemanding, thanked everyone a million times, said 'sorry' a lot for no reason and faded into the background, away from the beady eye of the hospital bed manager).

A side room is the ideal hosting location. During the evening, when there are hardly any doctors milling about, I think you could get away with a full-blown party. Tonight, my friends are desperately trying to persuade me to host my first hospital gathering.

'I can't let them come.' I pass my phone to Mum, showing her the messages.

'Why not? You're doing so much better now, Tilly.'

'Are you serious?' I snap. 'Look at me.'

I gesture down to the bruises covering my skin, the cannulas poking out of the creases in my arms, the drip pumping meds into my veins, the multicoloured wires stuck to my chest.

Mum moves from her chair and squishes up to me on the bed. I feel bad for snapping.

'Tilly, these are your best friends. They *want* to come. They've arranged a whole plan to get here because they love you.'

I begin to pick at my cuticle, a gross habit I've developed in moments of stress. I shred a bit of skin from around my thumbnail. A blob of blood seeps out and trickles down my hand.

'Hey, stop that,' Mum says, handing me a tissue.

I press it into my skin.

'I don't want them to see me like this.' I turn my head away and stare at the wall, tracing my eyes over the cracks in the plaster and crumbling paintwork.

'They won't ever really understand if you don't let them in.'

I keep staring ahead.

'You decide, Tilly. It's up to you.'

She moves back to the chair. I instantly wish she'd come back. I want her to look me in the eye and tell me exactly what to do; and yet, I know that if she does I'll proceed to argue every reason as to why she's wrong. Basically, Mum can't win. Actually, nobody can win. When people text saying, 'I don't want to bother you . . .' I feel like screaming, 'I *want* to be bothered!' I want them to drop me a text or a card. It hurts when they don't, when their own lives take over and I'm stuck watching it all unfold from the sidelines. And yet now, they are bothering a bit *too much*.

I try telling them I'm not feeling well enough but they aren't backing down.

A separate message pops up from Finn.

Go on Tills . . . everyone misses you!

I turn to Mum, the flicker of a smile now visible.

'Right, we better get out the hairbrush and dry shampoo,' I say.

She joins me on the bed again.

'I'm going to suggest something totally wild,' she begins. 'How about you go all out and have a *shower*?'

I can hear my friends' voices down the corridor, punctuated by Finn's, 'Shh, shh . . .' as he guides them into my room, presumably trying to draw as little attention as possible to the six visitors descending on the ward at once (the maximum of two per bed can be stretched a bit when you have a side room; this is less a rule and more down to the fact that nobody can see you).

My hair is washed. I have a clean set of loungewear on and Mum has sprayed me in her trademark perfume. I'm as ready as I'll ever be to invite my friends into my other world, the one I usually try to keep strictly separate.

Pia, Bella and Rosie bustle in first, followed by Luke, Josh and Finn. We were all placed on the same staircase together in first year and have since then become quite the unit. They all share two qualities: they are always up for fun and each of them has a very big heart. For so long, they've tried to be there for me but I've kept pushing them away. Now, they cross the threshold into my hospital room and, for the first time, my two separate lives collide.

'Oh, Tilly, you poor thing,' Pia says, rushing over to embrace me in a hug. 'Oh no, the tubes – sorry, I haven't hurt you, have I?'

'Don't worry, the cannulas are pretty bendy.'

She looks at me blankly. I realise she has no idea what a cannula is. I mean, fair play, why should she?

Finn sits beside me, holding my hand. The girls perch at the end of the bed and Luke and Josh each pull up a chair.

'And how are *you*?' Bella turns to Mum. 'Can we do anything to help you?'

Bella's sister has spent a lot of her life in and out of hospital, so she knows what it's like watching someone you love being poorly. She always properly asks how Mum, Dad and Finn are doing. I love her for it.

'I'm fine, Bella, I'm fine – but thank you for asking,' Mum smiles.

'Why don't you go and have a break?' Bella says. 'We can look after Tilly.'

'Are you sure you don't mind?' Mum asks.

'Of course,' Bella says.

Mum eventually agrees and begins gathering some of her things.

'Where are you going to go?' Luke asks.

'Ooh, Luke, I'm off for a big night out with Tilly's dad at . . . the hospital cafe,' Mum laughs.

'The hospital version of a big night out,' I grin.

We all wave her off and I immediately want to dive into everything I've missed.

'That's irrelevant. How are you feeling, Tilly?' Rosie interrupts.

'I'm good.' I'm obviously not good. I have pneumonia. Again. No one knows why and while the IV antibiotics have, as always, dampened it down, the window of time they work for is getting shorter and shorter. I'm actually pretty scared. Tonight, though, I don't want to think about any of that.

'It could be worse,' Josh says, gesturing around the room. He's spot-on. It could, and usually it is – so much worse. Tonight, my friends are seeing the sort of hospital setup they show on TV, when politicians occasionally grace the wards with their presence. It's all about giving the *impression* of perfection, kind of like I'm doing now. I have my own room, hidden away from the sights, sounds and smells of other patients. Mum has cleaned it so thoroughly it's practically gleaming. Part of me wants to say, 'No, no, you've got it all wrong, this isn't what hospital's *really* like,' and another part wants them to believe that this is how it is. It feels less scary letting them in this way.

'So, are you better?' Luke asks.

It's a reasonable question, I suppose, and one that makes sense the first time someone's ill, but I never really know how to answer.

'For now,' I smile and with that swiftly change the subject.

For a couple of hours, we chat and laugh. This is the world I want to be immersed in 24/7, but at 8pm Mum and Dad return and it's time for my guests to leave. The others step outside to give me a few minutes with Finn on my own.

'I know you weren't sure about everyone coming . . .' Finn begins. I frown and pull a mock-annoyed face. 'But I feel like maybe you actually kind of enjoyed it?'

'I did. I really did,' I smile. 'I hate to admit it but maybe you were right . . . Not that this is becoming a regular occurrence.'

'Definitely not, because in the future you being in hospital won't be a regular occurrence.' Finn squeezes my hand.

I fiddle with my hospital wristband. He's wrong. It's becoming more regular than ever.

'Everyone was so excited to see you. It's not the same without you,' he says. I look up at him, unsure what to say. 'I love you,' he whispers.

They say falling in love for the first time is the best feeling in the world. I'd add that when you have a chronic illness, it is also the most stressful. Finn is constantly offering to hop on trains and buses and bikes, to trek to whichever hospital I'm in, even just to see me for half an hour. I'm constantly saying no. Each time, I can hear the hurt in his voice and yet I'm convinced that what will hurt him more is seeing too much of this horrible hospital life. I'm frightened that it will seep into our happy life together and ruin the one great thing that we have.

After a few minutes, Bella pokes her head around the door.

'Finn, we need to head . . .'

He drops a brief kiss on my lips.

'You'll be back with us soon, Tilly.'

They all wave through the gap in the door. Then, the door swings closed and they are gone. They can continue the banter all the way home. I have to stay here, in bed, feeling like crap, watching from the sidelines. And yet, as the room empties, I am the one consumed with guilt.

'Finn could have a girlfriend who's well, who's there all the time, who can do all the things he wants to do,' I say to Mum and Dad.

'That's not how it works.'

'Finn wants to be with *you*,' Dad says.

'When you love someone, you love them. You can't just switch off loving them because they're ill or because something changes,' Mum agrees.

I circle my finger around the mottled purple bruise spreading across my forearm.

'The Tilly he loves is so much more than all of this.' She gestures around the sterile room.

It's hard to even picture the other girl, the Tilly that exists outside of all of this – but tonight, for just a couple of hours, I did snatch a glimpse of her.

Last night, I was effectively hosting a hospital gathering. Now, I'm once again bent over a cardboard sick bowl, retching. My whole body is furiously shaking. My teeth are chattering together so hard they sound like they could crack but I can't stop them. My hair is wet with sweat and the searing pain in my right lung is making me squeal out each time I breathe in. *If my friends could see me now.*

'Where's your call-bell?' Mum starts rifling through the sheets. It turns out it has somehow got wrapped around my T-shirt and is hanging over my shoulder. She presses it. Then, we wait and we wait and we wait. Nobody comes.

'Right, I'm just going to stand at the door and try to get someone, Tilly.'

Mum proceeds to hover by the door, one foot in my room, one out in the corridor. Her eyes ritualistically follow each member of staff as they walk past. The staff are like fish in an aquarium. There isn't a moment where they can just go about their business, undisturbed. Every second of their day they are watched and monitored by anxious patients and visitors. The doctor takes a step from left to right; our heads turn from left to right. The doctor disappears; our necks stretch to see where he's gone. A doctor we recognise emerges on the ward; our eyes are glued to her, hopeful that she's here to help us. We all want their attention but there aren't enough of them to go around.

Mum finally manages to make eye contact with a nurse. She says she'll get a doctor. Half an hour later, we're still waiting. Mum rings my call-bell again. Nobody comes.

She resumes her position at the door.

'Sorry, I'm so sorry, but I was told about half an hour ago a doctor would be coming to see my daughter Tilly. She's really deteriorated since last night.'

'We're really busy today. Three of the nurses are off sick and we're down to two doctors,' a nurse tells her.

'Sorry. I do, of course, understand. If you could maybe just mention that we're still waiting?'

The nurse nods and walks off. The pressure in the fishtank is building. It is ready to burst.

An hour later, a doctor rushes in. She's called Emma. I recognise her as one of the juniors on the respiratory team. She was standing behind the consultant on the ward round this morning.

'It's so busy out there today,' Mum says. 'It must be a nightmare for you all.'

Emma takes a breath and flattens her hair.

'It is, it is. I am so sorry to keep you waiting, Tilly.'

No one ever says sorry. I instantly like her.

'Now, what's going on?'

Mum begins to explain how I've started to go downhill.

'We don't understand it, she was really picking up. She even had some of her friends to visit last night.'

Emma nods.

'I did notice you didn't seem very well this morning. I actually brought it up with my seniors at our team meeting earlier.'

'Oh, thank you, thank you so much,' Mum says. 'She's got much worse since you saw her.'

I just sit there shaking, letting the conversation float over me.

'They took down one of the IV antibiotics, you see,' Emma says. 'I wondered if that could be why.'

I turn my head upwards to Emma, unable to conceal the panic on my face.

'They've taken one down? What do you mean?' Mum says, looking up at the drip next to me.

'We had Tilly on two types of antibiotics but they decided her X-ray was normal, so my consultant removed one.'

'Nobody told us that.'

It makes so much sense now.

'I'm worried she's not in a good place.' Mum gestures down to me.

'I agree with you. I actually thought I could see something on her X-ray but my seniors said it was normal, so they haven't had it reported on. I can't contradict my seniors . . .'

She pauses for a moment.

'So, what do we do?' Mum asks.

When you've lived with an illness for so long, you become the expert no one wants to be. I know when the pneumonias are taking hold. I know when I need the IVs. I also know that familiar feeling when I don't get them. The sweats, shivers, sickness, cough are all obviously grim; but there's another feeling, which is totally invisible to the eye. It's like there's anaesthetic running through my veins, drugging me and turning my body into a dead weight, so that even the motion of lifting my head feels like an effort. It's this feeling that continues to swamp me overnight and by the next morning has reduced me to an exhausted heap.

At 8am, there's a light tap on my door. Emma creeps in quietly and gestures for Mum to stand with her by the window. They talk in low, hushed voices but from where I lie, I can still hear what they're saying.

'You're here so early,' Mum says.

'I've just popped in before my shift begins. I was really concerned about Tilly last night.'

'Oh, Emma, that really is so kind.'

'My partner is actually part of the cystic fibrosis team at one of the top London hospitals. I hope you don't mind but I spoke to him about Tilly's case last night.'

'Of course not, I really can't thank you enough.'

'Now, as I told you yesterday, as a junior I can't override my seniors and ask for Tilly's X-ray to be reported on.'

Mum nods.

'I understand.'

'If, though – *hypothetically* – the patient or patient's family were to insist that it be reported on . . . Well, then we would be obligated to do it . . .' She raises her eyebrow, looking directly at Mum.

I like Emma's style.

The situation remains hypothetical for all of two seconds and then Mum officially asks to have the X-ray reported on. Emma documents this in the notes, then returns to her seniors and tells them that the patient's family have insisted. Fast-forward 24 hours, my X-ray is reported on. It turns out Emma is right. I have pneumonia. The second IV antibiotic goes back up. I begin to get better.

Before we leave the hospital, Mum calls Dad.

'I need you to pop to the shops and buy something for this lovely junior doctor.'

Dad laughs.

'So, what do we think this Emma would like, then?'

We decide what Emma would very much like is a box of Belgian chocolates. We attach a little note:

You are exactly the sort of doctor the world needs. Please, never change.

PATIENT SURVIVAL TIPS

- Invisible illnesses can be hard for people to understand. Sometimes they need to *see* what's really going on behind closed doors.
- 'I didn't want to bother you,' people will say. Tell them you *want* to be bothered. A card, text or call shows that someone out there cares.
- Love isn't a switch that can be turned on and off. The people around you love *you* for *you*.
- If, as a patient or family member, you insist that something needs to be done, ask for your request to be documented in writing (a paper trail is always a good idea).
- You should never underestimate a junior doctor (and neither should their seniors).

5

PERSPECTIVES

Post-discharge, I spend a few days resting up on the sofa. A week on, I am now desperately trying to persuade a reluctant Mum and Dad to take me back to Oxford.

'I just don't think you're well enough,' Mum keeps saying.

After a few tearful outbursts from me, Dad caves.

'Well, maybe let's just take her back and we can always come and get you if anything happens, Tilly,' he says. 'We're just a phone call away.'

'Yes, yes exactly. Listen to Dad.' I feel bad as I say this. It's a classic 'good cop, bad cop' scenario. Deep down, I know Mum is the one who is right here. I'm not well enough. The antibiotics just aren't working like they used to and there are already signs that the infection is rearing its ugly head again.

'You're an adult, Tilly, it's up to you. All I can tell you is what I think,' Mum says.

So, of course, I proceed to make the very unadult decision to head back.

*

The 'make Tilly move as little as possible' plan is fully underway and within a few hours of being back at university there is a familiar knock on my door. I peek around the quad, to check no one is watching, then surreptitiously take a large pile of books from Elliot. As arranged by my college, Elliot has been collecting my library books for over two years, thus saving me vital steps. Yet, I still know nothing more about him than his first name. This stems only from fear. I dread a scenario where Elliot hangs around too long and my friends spot him and realise what he's doing. It's best we remain total strangers.

I pull out this week's reading list and trace my finger down the texts. This term my special paper is focused on my favourite author, Virginia Woolf. I pick up my copy of *A Room of One's Own*, the text that inspired me to apply to Oxford. The concept of a woman needing a room of her own to write fiction really spoke to me. So many other areas of my life were and continue to be restricted but I have always been able to sit in my room and write. Studying requires no movement. It is the one thing I can do from the sofa. For years, reading has become my escape. Thinking about it, my parents must be delighted – 'How does your daughter cope with all of this?' 'Oh, she reads . . .' In the scheme of my life, if books are my only 'vice', I'd say I'm doing pretty well.

I look out across the beautiful college quad. Rain is trickling down the panes of my bay window and yet, even on this dullest of days, it remains magical. There really could not be a more motivating place to write. I check the time. It's now 1pm. That's five hours ahead of me before dinner. Over the years, I've had to train myself to be totally focused. When I'm working, I am 100 per cent working. I often have sleepless nights, which means lying in during the morning, so my window for getting things done is simply smaller than everyone else's. Getting distracted isn't an option. While my body may be failing, my mind still works; and for the next five hours I don't move from my desk.

After dinner, the familiar sharp pain begins searing through my right lung. *You shouldn't have come back. You know you shouldn't have come back.* I try to push the thought away.

Later, Finn swings by and, for the first time in weeks, we finally have some alone time together. I lie on the bed and press my body into his, leaning against his chest.

'It's so good to have you back, Tills. I've missed you.' He kisses the top of my head.

This sends a rush of panic through my body. *I'm not going to be back for long.*

The more lovely things he says, the worse I feel. It's like a pressure building up inside. My right lung burns. I clench my jaw. I can't let him see how unwell I'm feeling. I do what I have done for too long; for a few hours I perform the role of the 'perfect' girlfriend. I tell Finn what I think he wants to hear.

'How are you feeling?' he asks.

'Yes, better,' I lie.

'You still have your cough.'

I shrug it off and change the topic. We lie and chat and then put on a series we'd been watching together before I left, which he's saved for my return.

Three episodes later, he sits up.

'I think you need a proper night's sleep tonight, so I'm going to head off,' he says. 'But it's great to have you back.'

My heart sinks. I'm living a lie. Within seconds of him leaving I crash onto the bed, hug my body tightly in my arms and let it all out. I cry and I cry. There is only so long you can act for. At 3am, my lung pain intensifies. I begin to shiver and my teeth chatter together; 'rigors', they call this in hospital. Whenever I get the rigors I know things aren't looking good. At 3:15am, I make the call.

'I need you to come and get me,' I whisper down the phone to Mum.

'We'll be straight there, Tilly. Dad's grabbing the keys right now.' And because Mum is a real-life angel, she never once says, 'I told you so.'

This week, I was due to have tutorials on Chaucer, Rossetti and Woolf. Swap Chaucer for a chest X-ray, Rossetti for resus and Woolf's *A Room of One's Own* for 'Never in a million years will you get a moment alone' and once again, I've unfortunately found myself in a very different kind of story – although one with an equally entertaining host of characters.

This morning, I am awoken not by Elliot knocking on my door to deliver piles of canonical literature but by Margaret, on the phone to her friend Rita, at 5am.

'Oh, did I wake you, love?' Margaret booms down the phone. 'Just thought it would be nice to have a catchup.' There's a moment's pause. 'I CAN'T HEAR YOU, LOVE. One second, let me put you on loudspeaker.'

Is she for real?

By 5:30am, in between chesty coughs and rasps for breath, I have learned that Margaret is awaiting a lung transplant, is furious that her niece Lisa hasn't visited – 'The cheek of it, after all I've done for her' – and thinks the hospital tea tastes like 'dishwater' (very fair). Thanks to the loudspeaker function (or *malfunction*), I have also learned that Rita is extremely worried about Margaret, thinks Margaret should 'disown' Lisa and that when Rita had her hip replacement last year, she befriended a healthcare assistant called Mario, who not only had a 'gorgeous face' but also made a 'killer cup of tea'.

'SHUT UP!' a voice booms from Bed 4 opposite.

'Ooh, Rita, I think I've woken up one of the ladies.'

'Turn off the speaker!' the same voice yells.

'No need to lose your marbles, love,' Margaret shouts back, chuckling to herself.

We are all losing our marbles – including Rita's husband Fred, who we've heard has been 'moaning' at her for the last half an hour for keeping him awake. Fred could, presumably, escape his wife and move into another room. We, on the other hand, are trapped.

'Calm down, Fred, poor Margaret is in hospital.'

Our nurse, Dennis, enters the bay.

'NURSE! NURSE! This lady keeps using the phone on speaker, so early!' Bed 4 shouts.

Dennis is now a little stuck. I'm sure he can see it isn't ideal hospital etiquette to take calls in the middle of the night, but he doesn't have the power to actually stop Margaret or confiscate her phone.

'It is a bit early, my dear,' he begins. 'Some poorly people are trying to sleep.'

'Oh, Rita, my nurse sounds like your Fred.'

'Maybe you could chat a bit later?' Dennis politely poses.

'YES! So the rest of us can sleep!' Bed 4 chips in again.

'Or maybe we could turn off the speaker?'

'But then I can't hear Rita . . .'

The tension is building. I'm foreseeing Dennis breaking up a full-blown fight as catheters and cannulas fly through the air.

Eventually, it is Rita who makes the call to hang up, insisting she doesn't want to get Margaret into the 'naughty books'.

I think it's a little late (slash early) for that, Rita.

A message pings through from Finn.

How are you doing?

I quickly type a response:

I'm OK. On IVs again. Think maybe I just didn't have them for long enough before. I'll call you later x

Then I quickly turn my phone screen-down. I can't face seeing his response yet. I just want to shut it all out.

A few hours later, Dr Thomas pokes his head around the curtain, ready to begin the morning ward round. A queue of juniors shuffle in behind him.

'This is quite an interesting case: repeated pneumonia, emergency bowel resection. No known cause . . .' The juniors nod but continue to look down at their hands. 'She was only discharged last week but the infection has already returned. Looks like this IV antibiotic is starting to work now. Strong stuff but it's becoming less effective each time we use it.'

He finally turns to me.

'So, a few days of this and then I think you can head home again.'

'I really want to go home.' I'm always sure to state this, to overcome the common misconception that patients *want* to be in hospital. It's an assumption that always confuses me. Just look around – why would anyone *want* to be here? 'But the problem is, I'll just be back. No one has worked out why the pneumonias keep happening.'

Twice in two weeks is a new record.

'Sometimes in medicine, Tilly, we don't find the cause.'

It would help if anyone was looking. Over the last few weeks, I've seen so many different doctors. Each one has ordered another bag of antibiotics and headed off. When I ask if they can think of any reason why I keep getting pneumonia, the same answers reel off their tongues like a script: 'Oh, that's above my pay grade . . .' 'I couldn't comment, that's not my discipline . . .' 'I wouldn't like to muddy the waters . . .'

Please muddy the waters, *please*. I *need* someone to muddy the water. The only person trying to muddy the waters is Mum, who had to leave school with no qualifications and has no medical background. Mum is always *thinking*. It's heartbreaking to see just how much of her life is now confined to her laptop screen, endless days and nights buried in medical research papers.

'We sometimes reach a stage where we have to say to patients there is nothing left to investigate but what we can do is help you to manage the symptoms. How does that sound?'

It sounds a lot like giving up.

'You can try lifestyle moderations like doing more exercise, eating lots of fruit and vegetables – and it's really important to set little goals, to stay motivated.'

If this is the person currently managing my case, I am quite literally screwed.

'But exercise makes the pneumonias more frequent and I've been told to go on a low-fibre diet ever since my bowel resection . . .'

Let's not get onto motivated. I'm trying to do an Oxford degree from a hospital bed.

'Those were just examples.'

'Right, but if the antibiotic tablets aren't stopping the infections anymore and the strongest IV you can use is becoming less effective, where does that leave me, Dr Thomas?'

He doesn't answer.

'Dr Thomas, obviously I'm not a doctor . . .' *Good start from Mum.* 'But I do spend a lot of time researching and I do have a few suggestions of tests that, in my understanding, still haven't been done.'

'Like what?'

'My documents are at home but my first question would be:

does Tilly have an infection or could she have inflammation? I understand *both* respond to antibiotics.'

He gives her a sideways glance.

'Hard to tell.'

'Has anyone looked into Familial Mediterranean fever or cystic fibrosis or IgG deficiency or adult-onset mitochondrial disease . . .?'

Dr Thomas puts his hand up in the air, gesturing for Mum to stop.

'Very unlikely to be those, very rare.'

'After all these years of searching, is it not likely to be something very rare, Dr Thomas?' Mum smiles a friendly yet assertive smile.

'Well, we're not going to solve that today. Anyway, we've got lots of other patients to see now . . .'

Mum isn't willing to let up.

'Well, if you'd be open to having a look, maybe I could bring some of my documents in from home?'

'Yes, erm, yes OK, Mum.'

She's not your mum. She has a name.

With that, he slides out of the curtain.

And with that, I crumble.

There is so much talk, these days, about living in the present moment – but what happens when your present is torture? I look down at the scuffed white plasters lining my arms, the knobbly green cannula sticking out of the fine, raw skin on my hand and the gooey grey glue marking my chest in circular dots, where the ECG was applied. This isn't the present I want. I *have* to live in the future.

The future that usually exists in my mind offers hope that things will change, that I will get better. Today, it feels like Dr Thomas has snatched that hope away.

'I'm going to be left to die.' My voice cracks and tears begin to spill down my cheeks. It's rare that I have a full-on outburst but these tears are unstoppable. Mum wraps her arms around me and holds me tight. I curl into a little ball, a wet tissue held to my runny nose, my tears staining the sheets and pillow.

'Not on my watch.' Mum holds my head in her hands and turns it so I am looking directly into her eyes. 'I will not let that happen, Tilly.'

'No one here is even interested in looking for it,' I splutter between hiccuping sobs.

'That is not true, Tilly. I am.'

I can't deny that. When I'm back home, it has become normal to wake in the morning to find Mum still in front of her laptop, taking all-nighters to a new level. I'm torn between overwhelming guilt at seeing even more of her life devoted to being my own personal medical detective and fear that if she doesn't keep doing this, a future of ambulances, pain and hospital admissions is all that awaits me.

'Why do you do it?' I whisper.

'Because I'm a mum.'

'Not all mums would do this.'

'There's a reason why you suddenly became poorly, Tilly. This isn't about *me* being right. This is about what *is* right. If they won't find it, I will.'

'I feel like it's hopeless.'

'Giving up is *never* an option, Tilly.'

I nod.

'If you give up, then I give up and we can't have that can we?'

I shake my head.

'Anyway, Dr Thomas has agreed to see my research . . .' Mum grins, nudging my shoulder.

I manage a brief smile.

'He was basically saying they're going to leave me to die.'

'Tilly, he was saying all sorts of things. He was telling you to do exercise and eat the wrong diet. He doesn't know you; and for that very reason we can't trust what he says.'

Mum makes a good point.

'Now, I'm just going to give Dad a quick ring to come and sit with you, as I need to go to sort my papers ready to present my case to Dr Thomas tomorrow morning.' She winks at me.

'He's not going to know what's hit him,' I say between my tears.

I lie still while Mum begins packing up her things. Dr Thomas is now talking to Margaret next door. I overhear that her lung transplant has been booked in for tomorrow.

'So, doctor, can I have a few ciggies tonight? Seems a shame not to make the most of the free pass before I get my new lung . . .'

'Smoking is the reason you need this transplant, Margaret. So, we'd strongly advise against that.'

He can't stop her, though. Margaret is, after all, an adult who can make her own decisions in hospital as in life.

Mum goes down to meet Dad at the main entrance.

'Guess who we saw?' she says when they return.

I point next door to Margaret's cubicle.

'Yes, having a cup of tea and . . .'

'A cigarette.' I finish her sentence.

Dad begins tutting in the chair beside me.

'You would quite literally do anything to get better.' He gestures next door. 'Think of all the time, resources, funding going into that lung and she's out there, in a hospital gown with a drip hanging from her arm, smoking.'

It's a visceral image that all too often crowds the front of hospitals. It makes me sad each time I see it. I think of a story my friend Jaz shared with me from her medicine interview. I pose it to Dad.

'Two people have broken their leg, Person A is a fit, healthy, non-smoker who went on a skiing holiday and fell down the mountain. Person B is a chain-smoker who tripped walking to work. You only have the resources to treat one patient – who do you treat?'

'Skiing's a bit different to smoking,' Dad says.

'But is it? Person A *chose* to do a *dangerous* sport. You could claim it's no different to *choosing* to smoke cigarettes.'

Dad pauses for a moment, mulling it over.

'Then you have to think, did Person B grow up in a family of smokers? Did they understand the dangers before they got addicted? Is it their *fault* they ended up in this position?' I pose.

'Well, when you put it like that, I'm starting to think I got poor Margaret all wrong.'

It is 9am the next day. A porter arrives ready to wheel Margaret out of our bay and down the corridor for her lung transplant.

At the same moment, Mum walks into our bay, wheeling a suitcase bursting with research papers. This morning, two people are being offered a second chance at life: one by medical science and one by a mother unwilling to give up on her daughter.

When Dr Thomas arrives in our bay, he looks from Mum to the suitcase and back to Mum again.

'You asked for my documents,' she smiles.

PATIENT SURVIVAL TIPS

- Loving someone sometimes involves saying the things they don't want to hear.
- 'Obviously I'm not a doctor . . .' Before putting forward any of your (highly researched) patient opinions, get this phrase in. 'Google doctors' can be some medics' worst nightmare.
- Sharing your situation with someone who *really* knows you may give you a new perspective.
- If something doesn't add up, do your own research.
- TURN OFF your loudspeaker.

PATIENT SURVIVAL TIPS

6

FIGHT

Dear Tilly,

I am writing to inform you that due to the 6-week residency rule at the University of Oxford, you are now required to take a year out and return to your studies when you are able to meet the residency and course requirements.

I read and reread the email, certain that I must have misinterpreted it. The relentless determination and work I put into reaching Oxford has made me savour every moment. It continues to give me a facet of identity beyond the 'patient', allowing me to be a 'student' and to occupy a world full of opportunity and promise, so distinct from the other part of my life. This goal has remained my unwavering focus. It's a positive distraction, a motivation – and also means I'll have something to show for a time when it would have been so easy to give in. Once I have my degree, no one can ever take it away.

I race into the kitchen to break the news to Mum and Dad. We pull the email up on my laptop.

'I didn't even know there *was* a residency rule,' I say.

We calculate that they're right: I've now missed six weeks out of an eight-week term. But I've never fallen behind. I've completed Old English translations in waiting rooms, dissected Virginia Woolf on wards and, only earlier today, I emailed my tutor, Elena, with two assignments I'd caught up on this week.

'A year out isn't going to help me. I'm not getting better, only worse.'

I see my words slice through Mum and Dad, the hurt visible in their eyes. I'm saying the very thing none of us want to admit. We've heard no news from Dr Thomas since Mum presented her papers. With no medical teams actively trying to uncover the cause, I'm stuck on a conveyor belt destined to keep taking the same route. I'm the abandoned suitcase at the airport. If no one claims me, I'll be condemned to a future in 'lost luggage', forgotten and ignored. A year off doesn't offer a solution; it just furthers the torment along the way.

'There will be a way to sort this, Tilly. We'll find a way,' Mum says.

I head up to my room and stare out of the window. Thick grey nimbus clouds loom down from the sky. The grass outside is wet and boggy. A tear streams down my cheek. I call Finn.

'Always smiling' – that's what people say about me and that's how I want it to stay, but somehow it feels easier to let Finn into this, something practical, something more tangible than the illness, which is just so hard to explain. Much of the time, I live in an unreachable zone, a place so far removed that he can't relate. And yet, the news that I might have to take a year out of university, Finn can understand. He can relate to it because this is the world he occupies.

'It's all because of some ridiculous rule,' I say.

'Rules are there to be broken, Tilly,' he responds.

I can hear shouting from the kitchen. I creep downstairs and sit on the bottom step.

'This is adding a layer of stress she doesn't need. Maybe she *should* be taking a year out.' Dad's voice.

'I know that more than anyone. I'm the one dealing with it day in day out,' Mum responds.

'I understand that but I have to work.'

'Work is nothing compared to this.'

'That's not what we were discussing. We were talking about whether this degree is too much, and I think it is at the moment.'

'OK, so she gives it up. Then what does she have?' Mum poses.

'She has time to rest, time to recover.'

'She said it herself: she's *not* recovering. Right now, she's *not* recovering and a year out isn't going to help that.'

'Don't say that. Stop saying that.' I can hear the pain in Dad's voice.

'OK, you just bury your head in the sand. You do that while the rest of us face up to what's really happening here.'

'That's unfair. I just think the stress can't be helping her.'

'I think the opposite. This degree is what's keeping her going.'

I walk in then and take in the sight of my parents, both of them exhausted and weary. I know how much they try to hold it together for me, but sometimes we all need to let it out. A look of sadness passes between them, as they realise I've heard every word that's been said. Stress binds us but it also tears us apart.

'I'm sorry, Tilly. You shouldn't have to hear this,' Dad says. 'What's your view?'

'I think wrapping me in cotton wool and stopping me from living isn't the answer.'

When I wake the next morning, I find Mum in the same position on the floor, surrounded by pieces of paper and reams of notes.

'I've found it!' she exclaims. 'It's taken all night but I've found it.' She points to the large book of my university's rules and regulations, which has so far only ever been used as my doorstop. 'There's a precedent here of a student who extended from a three-year to four-year degree, instead of taking a year out.'

I let out a cheer and fling my arms around her. Spreading my degree over a longer period of time to account for hospital admissions makes so much more sense. Mum embraces me in a tight hug, then leans her head back against the wall, her body crumpling into an exhausted heap.

'They can't argue with their own book,' she says.

'I don't know what I would do without you, Mum.' I squeeze her hand, noticing how fragile and thin it feels.

Guilt courses through me. This illness began as a light wind, rustling a few areas of my life, knocking a few things out of place, but it has since erupted into a tornado, ripping through everything – and everyone – that surrounds me.

*

After a few intense days of preparing my case, I walk into the quad ready for my meeting with the academic director. I keep telling myself this is what I'm good at; I've been fighting most of my life.

It's a miserable, grey day but the stone walls envelop me with their familiar warmth. Not only is it architecturally breathtaking but it also evokes a kind of magical quality I've never experienced anywhere else. I can't let them take this away from me.

At 5pm I'm led into the academic director's office. The welfare officer is sitting beside her, alongside my tutor, Elena. They smile at me as I enter but the atmosphere feels tense.

'How are you feeling?' Elena asks.

The truth is I'm feeling terrible. My cough is already returning and I know it won't be long before my body begins to spiral again. For today, though, my makeup is on, a smile is printed firmly on my face and I am not giving them any sign of weakness. I just need to get through this meeting and two weeks of term and then I can either regroup or end up in hospital. Welcome to my messed-up reality.

'I'm doing a lot better, thank you.'

With pleasantries out of the way, the meeting begins. The academic director opens by explaining the residency rule and course requirements and why it is necessary, in circumstances like mine, for students to take a year out to get better.

I understand the sentiment. If a student is ill once, they can give in to the process knowing that a year out of resting up will lead to a quicker recovery. They know that their stint as the patient has an end point. But what happens when there is no end in sight? What happens when your daily life is a constant cycle of appointments, prescriptions, admissions, procedures and emergencies? How long do you put your life on hold for?

I spend the next hour putting my case forward: the case that shows I don't fit the textbook definition of an 'unwell student'. It seems they've never had a student effectively break the news that they're not getting better. It's a sad story that I tell matter-of-factly, as if I am talking about someone else. This kind of self-protection proves the only way to get through.

Elena turns out to be my best ally. Before my cohort met her last term, her reputation as the 'dragon' preceded her. She was known for her harsh feedback and tough tutorials. Elena is tall, with a strong jawline and steely glare. She appears unbreakable. I was shocked when Pia messaged me earlier this term to tell me Elena had been diagnosed with cancer. I look at the wispy strands of grey hair now smattering her head. The chemotherapy has visibly taken its toll on her body and yet, her spirit remains. Today, she fights like a dragon for me.

The meeting ends with the academic director telling me she will look into the four-year degree, which she had never heard of before. She promises to get back to me by the end of term. It feels like a small win.

'Let's go to the SCR,' Elena says as we leave the office. 'You look cold.'

This time last week, I was lying in a hospital bed, connected to a drip. Now, I'm sitting in front of a roaring fire in the senior common room, its oak-panelled walls adorned with historic portraits, sipping coffee with my Oxford English tutor. I occupy two distinct worlds, so far apart they feel impossible to reconcile.

'I don't know how to thank you, Elena. Really, it means so much that you fought for me in there.'

She waves her hand, brushing it off as nothing.

'I didn't even know you were unwell when I met you last term,' she says.

'Ditto,' I reply.

'That's how I like it to be,' she responds.

'Me too,' I nod. 'Me too.'

A week later, I'm sitting in the library desperately refreshing my emails when one pops up with the subject line 'Extenuating circumstances'. I inhale. This is the news I've been waiting for. I scan through the opening sentences, focusing in on the only bit that matters.

I DON'T HAVE TO TAKE A YEAR OUT! MY FOUR-YEAR DEGREE HAS OFFICIALLY BEEN APPROVED!

There it is, in black and white: a paragraph plainly stating that I'll have the same number of tutorials, classes and lectures as my 'peers' but be given the time to make up for my 'absences' due to hospital admissions. It feels like the smoke that has been billowing around me, concealing the path ahead, has evaporated. I now have a future to hold onto. There's only one person truly responsible for my change in fate. I immediately pick up the phone to call Mum.

'I'll never know how to thank you for everything you do for me,' I say to her.

'I don't need thanking. The only thing I need is for you to get better.'

It's what everyone needs. I visualise myself at the centre of this thick smog, suffocating everyone in my wake. Lately, Mum and Dad seem to be constantly arguing. I know they love each other and I know they love me but they're both exhausted and starting to crumble. Finn desperately wants to be there for me but I'm so determined not to let this illness contaminate our relationship together that I keep pushing him away. When I'm with him and my friends I want to step outside the smog and escape for a few gulps of fresh air. My friends don't say much but I know they don't really understand. Invisible illnesses are confusing: 'Why can she go out tonight but not tomorrow?' 'Why does she keep bailing?' 'How can she be that ill when she looks fine?'

It feels like a contradiction. I've spent years trying to shake off the 'illness' label. I want to be just 'Tilly', not 'Tilly the patient', but without a label it's difficult for people to understand. Humans use names, labels and categories for structure and meaning. Without them, the world would be chaotic. Diagnostic labels in medicine work in the same way. Without a diagnosis, I'm floating in the clouds, suspended in the chaos of the unknown. I don't know why climbing the stairs everyday equals pneumonia. I don't know why I can head out Friday night but end up in A&E on Saturday. I don't know why my tummy is growing again or why I keep losing weight. I don't know why I am constantly breaking out in sweats and shivers. And not knowing is the worst bit of all.

PATIENT SURVIVAL TIPS

- Being a patient doesn't mean giving up on your dreams and goals. It means finding new ways to achieve them.
- Patient life is stressful. Sometimes it helps to get it off your chest and clear the air.
- There is a difference between surviving and living. Be respectful of your body but seize life when you can.
- Find *your* person. That may be someone different at each stage of your journey.
- Keep your fighting spirit alive.

7

LABELS

I am back home for Christmas and already the infection is taking hold again. This evening, as I lie on the sofa, my eyes wander to the large oak tree outside the window. I know this oak tree well. For years, I have seen it blossom in spring with luscious green leaves that fade into burnt oranges and yellow ochres in autumn. Now, the leaves have fallen and its dramatic branches make a silhouette against the evening sky. I know things about this oak tree that no one else knows because I have spent so much (too much) of my life on this sofa. I know that the pigeons gravitate to the third branch from the top, I know that the trunk has a jagged chunk missing from the right-hand side and I know that it holds several delicate nests, carefully constructed by the winter robins. My friend Eve once told me that robins are messengers from loved ones who have passed away. I always think of my great-grandma Grace when the robins appear from the depths of the trees and dart across the garden. Maybe she's watching over me now.

Mum opens the lounge door, concern etched into her face.

'Tilly, I have Dr Phillips on the phone.'

It takes me a moment to realise who she means. I liked Dr Phillips.

She was one of the consultants on the respiratory team during my last admission. I saw her only a couple of times but on both occasions she asked questions about *me*, the person beyond the patient. I remember her telling me how much she was missing her little girl, who had just started nursery. She was human.

I drag my hand up to my neck and attempt to shake my head, signalling that no, I feel too unwell, I do not want to talk to Dr Phillips. I point my finger at Mum, mouthing, 'You.'

Mum nods. We work in a code, an unspoken language I don't have with anyone else. It sometimes feels like Mum is an extra limb on my body, so much a part of me that we know what the other is thinking at any given time.

'Tilly really isn't feeling very well. Would you mind speaking to me on her behalf?'

Mum puts the phone on loudspeaker.

'I'll need to speak to Tilly – unless of course she gives permission for me to speak to you.'

I nod. Mum places the phone under my chin.

'This is Tilly. Please speak to my mum,' I murmur, flopping my head back onto the cushions. It makes me cough, a thick, crackling cough. I watch the beads of sweat pop through the skin on my legs and know that it won't be long until I'm back on the ward.

Mum leaves the room but the door is ajar. I can hear the conversation coming from the hallway.

'Sorry, I know it's late on a Friday night, but I had to call you before the weekend . . .' I miss the next bit. She says something about a 'QuantiFERON Gold test'.

What's that?

'The suitcase . . . your documents . . . fight my seniors for the test.'

I think of Mum wheeling her suitcase into the ward. *What test?*

'They said . . . would have already been tested.'

For what? I'm now leaning my head off the sofa, straining to hear.

'Tilly has tested positive for tuberculosis.'

Her words fly down the hallway, towards the sofa, catapulting me backwards with a force so strong it's tangible. *Tuberculosis? TB?* Is Dr Phillips saying I have TB? This makes no sense. How can I have TB? I pull the blanket up to my chin. Part of me wants to hide underneath it and never come out. Another part of me wants to hear every single word.

All I can think about is how I'm going to be labelled 'The Girl with TB'. That's how everyone will refer to me. TB's really infectious, isn't it? No one will want to come near me. My thoughts jump and dart and spiral into each other, blurring into confused and jumbled waves. I take a breath and try to compose myself. I need to hear what she's saying.

'White, middle-class . . . never travelled to any of the endemic countries . . . classic case . . . positive discrimination in medicine . . . doesn't fit the demographic.'

There is a pause.

'No one would have ever considered it.'

'How can Tilly have TB?' Mum's voice is steady but I can hear the undertone of fear.

'Was she vaccinated?'

'Erm no . . . no she wasn't. No, I remember, they'd actually stopped the vaccine by Tilly's year at school because . . . TB was eradicated . . . wasn't it?'

'It was but . . . more and more cases.'

Mum then asks the question swirling through my head.

'So, sorry, just to clarify, Dr Phillips, are you saying Tilly *has* tuberculosis?'

'It's a little complicated.'

I let out a breath. Maybe I heard it wrongly. Maybe it's not true.

'She has been infected with tuberculosis.'

Like a reflex, my cheeks clench and my eyes scrunch together. I place my hands over my face, as if by not seeing anything, her words will have less impact.

'But TB can either be *latent*, where you have been infected but it's dormant in the body; or it can be *active*, where it is actively giving you symptoms . . . need to work out which one Tilly has.'

'Right, right, OK, but Tilly *does* have symptoms. She's really poorly right now, Dr Phillips. The pneumonia is taking hold again.'

'Discuss properly . . . appointment . . . first thing Monday . . . deteriorates over weekend . . . must take her to hospital.'

Dr Phillips shares the appointment details. A few pleasantries are exchanged. Mum thanks her again and again, thanks her for testing me, thanks her for telling us that I have TB on her Friday night. So polite, even in the worst of times.

The silence beats through me as my mind registers what's just happened. Tears begin to spill from my eyes and within moments are pouring down my cheeks. I manoeuvre my body into a tight ball, with the blanket held up to my face, enveloping me in its soft wool. Mum walks into the room. She starts to speak.

'Tilly, I—'

'I heard it. I heard the whole conversation. I have tuberculosis.'

I don't think my Friday night can get any worse but then it does. I start vomiting, at the same time as shivering so hard my teeth are chattering; I'm dripping with waves of sweat, coughing up cement-like gunk and (excuse the detail) this all happens while sitting on the toilet because I now also have violent diarrhoea. My body is doing its thing again – where it sort of drags along for a while and then, without warning, grasps quite how ill it is and decides to show it through every bodily function. Nice.

At 5am on Saturday, Dad races through the empty roads to the hospital. On arrival at A&E, Mum has to tell them I have tuberculosis. She whispers this to the medical team and I sense them recoil slightly. It turns out, I was right: TB can be *highly* infectious. The only plus (and I mean *only*) is that I am assigned a side room. A side room on the oncology ward.

Oh yes, I know what would be a good idea: let's put the girl with raging TB on the ward with all the patients on chemo – all the patients with severely compromised immune systems.

Apparently, it's the only available side room in the entire hospital, and it's the most modern ward. A win for me; a massive blow for everyone else. Just to really panic the other patients, my door has a big sign with a red cross on it, saying, 'INFECTIOUS: DO NOT ENTER'. Below is a tick list of all the things the staff have to do before coming in. *Mask. Tick. Gloves. Tick. Apron. Tick.* I bet the nurses are out there playing fives to decide who has to enter.

It turns out Mum's wheelie suitcase, bursting with research, was just the sort of pressure Dr Thomas needed. He finally took my case to his team meeting. Luckily for me, the lovely Dr Phillips was in attendance. Mum's research built a case for looking at illnesses that respond to antibiotics and Dr Phillips had a brainwave about TB. She persuaded her reluctant seniors to do a test. They said I didn't fit the demographic, that I 'couldn't possibly have TB'. What a difference 24 hours can make. Now they all seem to think I have so much TB I'm spewing it over everyone I meet. Mum is the only visitor allowed in my room and even she has to wear a mask.

'We don't want you catching it, Mum . . .'

It hits me that if the staff here are that worried about me being infectious, just think how many people I could have infected out there. I look out of the window, making a mental list of all the people I've come into contact with; all the people who could now have TB *because of me*. I'm at the centre of a tight knot of wool. The people in my life are distinct strands of thread, now irrevocably ensnared in my messy spiralling ball. The more names I come up with, the bigger the ball grows.

'Finn's going to have TB,' I blurt out.

If I have TB, there is no way Finn *can't* have it. We've shared my tiny single bed pretty much every night of term for the last few years. (This was an error on my part. I invited him to stay in those first flushes of romance and then it became a habit – one that means he sleeps with half his body propped against the wall while I'm practically falling off the bed.) This sort of close proximity is surely prime TB-catching territory.

'I'm going to have ruined his life,' I sob. Imagine the family events:

'Hi, Aunt Edna, this is my girlfriend, Tilly. She has tuberculosis, so probably don't get too close.' I'm going to have to come with a warning sign. Finn's never going to sleep in that single bed again. He's going to find a lovely new girlfriend who isn't coughing up infectious disease over everyone she meets.

'Tilly, Tilly, stop letting your thoughts run away with you. We don't know anything for certain yet.'

My mind goes into overdrive. I decide that Mum, Dad and Finn definitely have TB. Then, surely, I'll have also given it to my friends. For so long, I've tried to keep the patient side of my life separate from them, imagining that if I didn't talk about it, it wouldn't contaminate our time together. Now I'm going to have to break the news that it lingers in the very air between us, something no words can block out.

Their families will be suggesting they stay away from me. I can hear it now: 'I wouldn't get too close . . .' 'I'd be a bit careful around her if I were you . . .' 'Steer clear, son . . .' One phone call and my whole life has changed. Waiting has always been one of the worst things about being a patient. I've been stuck in a perpetual waiting room, dependent on someone else calling my name. The lack of control over my own life has, at times, felt utterly futile; and yet it's a weird paradox, as the waiting part also holds possibility. For years, every night, I've quietly asked the universe for one thing: a diagnosis. Medical science relies on putting people in boxes. Without a label there is no cure. At last, my illness has a name but it's one I'm now desperate to hide: 'The Girl with TB'.

Mum puts on her assertive voice.

'Tilly, look at me.'

I refuse, continuing to stare out of the window. She carries on.

'You can't torture yourself with "what-ifs". Until you have the bronchoscopy on Monday, we don't even know you're infectious.'

I twist my head to look at her. In an act of rebellion, Mum pulls her face mask around her chin. She knows it's too late. I'll have already infected her. I'll have given Mum, the person I love most in the world, TB.

'They're making *you* wear a mask, *you*. They must think I'm infectious.'

The weekend is going by in a blur. Medical staff hurry in and out, just to change my cannulas and hook up new bags of antibiotics. When they take my blood pressure and pulse, I'm sure I can sense them pulling away, trying not to breathe in my air. They are distant, remote. No one stays to chat.

This morning, there's a light tap at the door and a lady walks in. She has long dark hair, tied back in a loose ponytail, and is wearing the same mask, gloves and apron as all of the others, but in her hand is a mop and bucket.

'Ooh, Tilly, I think your room's going to get a Sunday spruce,' Mum says.

I've met lots of hospital cleaners over the years but very rarely on a weekend and none like this lady. She scrubs the floor with energetic vigour until it gleams; she bends down using her weight to needle the dirt out of the windowsill; she grabs a chair and balances on it, stretching up to dust the ceiling; she smooths her hands over the taps again and again until they shine. By the time she's worked her magic in the bathroom, I would quite happily eat a Sunday roast off the toilet seat.

'OK?' She approaches the end of my bed and points to the remote control. It's covered in a series of buttons that can be used to change the shape of the mattress and move the bed up and down.

'Of course,' I say, not really sure what she's asking.

She proceeds to raise my bed up in the air, until I'm towering above the room. From up here, I can see out of the window towards the grey, concrete car park. I look across at the staff bays. During the week they are practically bursting. Today, they are virtually empty. A visible manifestation of the absurdity of the hospital rotas.

'Oh, wow, Tilly, your bed's getting the gold-standard clean.'

The lady glances up. Her eyes crease into a smile over her mask. She meticulously wipes her cloth along the metal bars at the side of my bed. Then suddenly, she is underneath my mattress, crouching down to clean the underside of my bed. Our eyes follow her every move.

'Tilly isn't allowed out and I've been staying with her.' Mum gestures to the bed, the cleanest bed there ever was. 'These things really do matter when you're stuck in here,' Mum says. 'What's your name?'

'Mrs Sarma,' she nods.

'Thank you, Mrs Sarma,' Mum says.

Mrs Sarma puts her hand up in the air and then leaves my room.

Five minutes later there's a tap at the door.

'Drink?' Mrs Sarma's head emerges through the gap.

Mum stands up and rushes towards her.

'Oh, a cup of tea would be wonderful.'

'Milk, sugar?' she whispers.

'Just milk, just milk,' Mum whispers back.

She nods and scurries off.

A minute later, the door opens enough for a gloved hand to stretch in, holding a steaming mug. Mum's eyes are dewy as she clasps it in her hands.

'Oh, Mrs Sarma, I always say: I can do anything as long as I have a cup of tea.'

PATIENT SURVIVAL TIPS

- Know that you can give consent in writing, in advance, or verbally, at the time, for someone to speak/advocate on your behalf.
- However many times you are told 'no', however many times you are told you must just 'accept' being ill, however many times you are not believed, never stop pushing for a diagnosis.
- Don't always just rely on one doctor; medicine is about opinion.
- This is *your* life. Do your own research. Knowledge can give you more control.
- Sometimes a cup of tea is enough to transform an entire day.

8

POWER

There's a knock at my door.

'I think the doctor's here,' I say down the phone to Finn.

'Will call you later.'

I am living a lie. I haven't yet told Finn about the TB. I'm afraid of what will happen if I do. Swap an 'infectious laugh' for 'actually infectious' and 'killer good looks' for 'I could actually kill you' and you have my dating profile. Not exactly goals.

Telling Finn would let him into a world I don't want him to be a part of; a world I can't control. Although, if it turns out I *am* infectious, I'll be forced to tell *everyone*. We've read online that for TB there is a process called 'contact tracing'. Think of it like selecting 'all contacts' in your phone and sending them a message:

> Hey there! Long time no speak. How are you doing? Would be great to catch up soon! Oh, and by the way, turns out I have really infectious TB and you may also have it. Mind popping to the doctor for a test? Tilly xoxo

Dr Phillips stands at the entrance to my room. The first thing I notice is that I can see her face. I look down at her body. She's not wearing an apron. She's not wearing gloves. *Does this mean . . .?*

Mum stands up.

'Please, sit down, sit down,' she says, gesturing to the hard, turquoise chair that has been her sofa, bed and office for the last five nights.

'No, no thank you,' says Dr Phillips. 'I have to rush off to pick up my little girl, but I couldn't leave without coming to tell you. We have the result of the bronchoscopy.'

I take a gulp, scared to look at her.

'Tilly, you aren't infectious.'

I let out a long, slow breath, pushing back my neck and turning my head up towards the ceiling. All week, I've been submerged in this sea of dread, desperately holding my breath, waiting, waiting for someone to return me to dry land. At last, I can breathe again.

The tight knot of wool that's been growing inside my tummy has now unravelled, as the people around me are set free. And yet, rather than feeling calm, my mind jumps onto the next fear, the one that I haven't had time to process because my brain has been too full. I can finally focus on the fact that I *do* have TB. There doesn't seem to be any uncertainty about that. What the doctors are now working out is which strain and what treatment I'll require. I think of that game 'Who Am I?' we sometimes play at family events, where each player has a Post-it note stuck to their forehead with a name on it and they have to guess who they are. A few days ago,

I was 'Tilly Rose' but my Post-it now reads 'The Girl with TB'. People won't see my smile, hear what I say or remember all the other facets of my identity. This label will define me. I want to rip the Post-it off and shred it into hundreds of tiny pieces.

There are so many thoughts, fears and worries to dissect but there's no time to reflect. This morning, the door never stops banging. Phlebotomists, nurses and doctors keep swinging by. By the afternoon, I'm exhausted. Just as I'm beginning to doze off, there's another knock – one that has now become familiar. Three rhythmic, light taps signal that Mrs Sarma is about to pay me a visit. She has popped by every day since we first met. She and Mum have communicated through a series of nods and smiles but mostly through cups of tea. Each morning before her shift begins, her gloved hand stretches through the doorway with a steaming mug. Mrs Sarma, and Mrs Sarma alone, has got Mum through the week.

'Oh, thank you. Thank you. A second cup today!' Mum exclaims. 'We've just found out some good news. Tilly definitely isn't infectious.'

Mrs Sarma looks puzzled. Mum points to the sign on my door with the big red cross and mimes drawing a line through it. Mrs Sarma puts her fists up in the air in a cheering motion and leans around my door, giving me a thumbs up. With that, she is gone.

'Right, now we're allowed out of the room, I might pop downstairs and make a few calls. Dad and Auntie have been ringing me all morning to check on you but it's been so busy, hasn't it?'

People often have this perception that patients spend their days lying in bed, bored out of their minds. Instead, we seem to spend most of the time running a research hub from the bed; hours spent googling away, making lists, improvising how we'll make the most out of our five-minute slot on the ward round to ask those all-important questions, agonising over how best to present our suggestions and thinking – so much brain space has been taken up thinking.

For the last week, every time I've stirred in the night, Mum's phone has been glowing in the chair beside me as she uses every spare moment to research. She always says that if she understands the science, then she can ask the right questions. I look over at her now, as she walks back into my room. Her eyes are tired. Her body is fragile. Our chapters together are bound by love; and yet guilt seeps across the pages like a smudged ink stain. This illness isn't just shaping my own narrative; it's forever changing the plots of those around me too.

'Tilly, I need to talk to you about something. I wish I didn't have to but I need to tell you this now, before the doctor comes.'

She sits down beside me and holds my hands in hers. I nod.

'I've just been on the phone to Grandma. I was explaining about the TB diagnosis and how none of us can understand how you could have it. Grandma mentioned our trip to Auntie Nora's farm when you were five.'

My great-aunt Nora owned a dairy farm in County Cork, Ireland. It was a five-year-old's holiday of dreams. Aunt Nora was the sort of farmer you'd draw as a child; she wore a faded floral apron, patterned with holes and stains. Her ginger perm was frizzy and the ruddy hue of her cheeks reflected a lifetime spent outdoors. Back then, I saw none of this, only that permanently on her feet were a pair of muddy wellington boots. My great-aunt made me breakfast in wellington boots. She quickly became my icon. Sadly, she passed away quite a long time ago, but I've always had such fond memories of that trip.

'I don't understand,' I say, urging Mum to go on.

'Well, Grandma said you would have drunk unpasteurised milk on that trip.'

I look at her, confused. *Unpasteurised milk?*

'OK . . .' I gesture for her to explain.

'Well, historically, lots of people used to get TB from unpasteurised milk,' Mum says.

'Wait . . .' I pause for a moment, mulling it over. It's too much to take in. 'So, you and Grandma think I got TB from drinking *unpasteurised milk* on Aunt Nora's farm?'

'I thought it was eradicated by the time you went to Aunt Nora's but Grandma said there have been odd cases. She said any milk you had back then on the farm would have been unpasteurised.'

I think back to that trip to Ireland; paddling in wild streams, hours spent running through wide open fields playing tag and hide and seek, and trotting through the woods, with my cousins, on horses that had no saddles. It was an adventure.

I stare ahead, numb and frozen.

'I'm sorry, Tilly, to have to tell you here like this.' Mum presses her hand tenderly against my cheek. 'But I've read there are different treatments for different strains of TB, so it's something I'm going to have to ask the doctor and I wanted to be able to discuss it with you first.'

Flashbacks of the farm, the TB result, my symptoms all compete in a frenzied dance in my mind, building in force, clamouring for my attention. I want to gather them up, lock them into little glass jars and place them on a shelf hidden from view, but I know these things never really go away. The jars will fill up and one day they'll overflow. So, I do what I have had to do so many times now: I allow myself a few minutes to consider it all, to feel the shock and sadness, and then I take a breath and pick Mum's brain on everything she has learned so far. She explains more about the two types of TB Dr Phillips spoke of on the phone: latent (dormant without symptoms) and active (with symptoms).

The more we read, the more we realise I have all the symptoms of *active* TB: recurrent pneumonias, lung pain, weight loss, night sweats, weakness, intestinal blockages. I can't believe it's never been tested until now. Mum goes on to explain about the different strains, the different treatment options and the potential sources of the infection.

'So, after all this time, you're saying a *cow* could have ruined my life?'

A few minutes later, there is another knock at my door.

'This is Dr Taylor,' I say to Mum. 'The doctor who did my bronchoscopy.'

He gives her a slight nod and then turns to me.

'So, you're not infectious,' he says. 'Knew you wouldn't be.'

I think of all the masks, gowns and gloves.

'Anyway, you have *latent* TB. It's unlucky but not responsible for your symptoms. With latent you have to take three months of drugs, so that it never activates in the future. We've already written up a prescription.'

'Sorry, so you're saying I definitely don't have *active* TB?'

He shakes his head.

'I have lots of the symptoms – pneumonias, cough, night sweats, terminal ileum resection, weight loss, no appeti—'

He cuts through before I can finish.

'And how long have you had these?'

'They started about 12 years ago.'

He laughs.

'You would be dead.'

I swallow.

'So, yes, I've instructed the nurse to prepare the latent drugs.'

'I'm a little confused. I thought patients with latent TB didn't have any symptoms. I have loads.'

Mum then repeats my list of symptoms, almost word for word. Dr Taylor turns his back, manoeuvring her out of the conversation.

'I am talking to the patient.'

He also has his back to his junior. It's as if she's not in the room.

'Can you speak to my mum please?' I whisper. It's too much to deal with. I just want to hide.

'I am talking to *you*.'

'Can I just . . .?' Mum tries to interrupt.

'*You* are the patient.' He twists his body to the side and faces me head-on, completely ignoring Mum.

'I'm Tilly's advocate,' Mum continues before he can answer, the words racing from her lips. 'I've just been on the phone to

Tilly's grandma and I was explaining about the TB and how none of us can understand how she could have it. Tilly's grandma said that when Tilly went to Ireland, aged five, she would have drunk unpasteurised milk on her great-aunt's dairy farm.'

Dr Taylor starts to shout.

'I've told you. You DO NOT have active TB. It's *not* the TB that is making you unwell.'

I recoil in the bed and tears start to well in my eyes.

'Please can you speak to my mum?' I say again.

'No, I am speaking to you. If you had active TB for this long, you would be dead.'

Mum leans forward in her chair to look up at him.

'Can I just check, then – just to placate me, Dr Taylor – does the QuantiFERON Gold test you have done test for *all* strains of TB, including bovine TB from unpasteurised milk?'

He rolls his eyes.

'No, it does *not* test for bovine. It's completely irrelevant that she has drunk the unpasteurised milk. Anyway, it's virtually eradicated. Nobody here gets TB from milk anymore.'

His face is now red, with a sweaty film across his forehead. Behind him, the junior sways from one foot to another, her gaze darting between Mum and the floor.

'She does *not* have active TB. She does *not* have bovine TB!' Dr Taylor shouts.

All week, so many elements of my life have been pulled from under me, shaking my very foundations. I know how important it is to stay strong, alert and logical in these conversations. I know that's the only way they'll listen to us, but Dr Taylor's words are grinding down the final layer of cement holding me together. I crumble.

The junior now tilts her head to look around him and directly at me. It seems it is possible to apologise with your eyes.

I look over at Mum, who is now wiping a tear from her cheek. Dr Taylor has managed to make my mum cry.

It's like a switch flicks inside him. He realises he's gone too far. Dr Taylor picks up a couple of tissues from my side table and hands one to each of us. He kneels down and holds onto the arm of Mum's chair.

'I can see you're finding it all quite overwhelming.'

'Can Tilly just have a little more time to think it all through before taking the latent drugs?' Mum asks.

He sighs.

'We really cannot wait too long.'

With that, he leaves the room.

I look over at Mum, usually so strong, upright, ready for battle. Dr Taylor has reduced her to a crumpled heap in the chair. She drops her head into her hand, her bony elbow resting on the hard wooden arm. I want to run after Dr Taylor. I want to scream and shout and ask why he would ever speak to anyone like that. I want to take him by the shoulders and shake him. Instead, I lie in the bed, weak and powerless. I stare ahead at the bare, white wall, mottled with patches of grey where the paint has peeled. I hate that I need him. I hate that he knows that. We interact as roles, not people. He is the doctor. I am the patient. Somewhere along the way, I have stopped being 'Tilly' in Dr Taylor's eyes.

PATIENT SURVIVAL TIPS

- Know that you have a year to register a complaint.
- If a treatment or diagnosis doesn't feel right, *question it.*
- *Everyone* is allowed an advocate.
- Medical results can be a lot to process; allow yourself a moment to *feel* and to consider your options before jumping into the next steps.
- You are *always* entitled to ask for a second opinion.

9

DETECTIVE

'Tilly, you can't start that treatment yet. I'm sure I've read that this QuantiFERON Gold tests for TB from milk,' Mum says.

'But Dr Taylor said that it doesn't.'

'But I'm sure I've read that it does,' Mum says.

'Surely he knows?' I look up at Mum.

'Nothing would surprise me anymore,' she shakes her head. 'People with latent TB don't have any symptoms. It just means it's in their body and they could develop it in the future. You have all of the symptoms. It's nonsense. It must be active.'

'Yes, but can I not just start the three-month latent course he was prescribing?'

'It doesn't work like that. Latent TB treatment is a three-month course, whereas active TB is at least a nine-month course and includes more drugs. I've read that if a patient takes latent drugs and they have active TB, then they can become drug resistant.'

'Like when you don't complete a full course of antibiotics?'

'Yes exactly,' Mum replies.

'So, if it turned out I did have active TB from milk, I'd probably just die because I'd have become drug resistant?'

'I won't ever let that happen.'

I return to my trance, staring up at the scuffed squares of grey inside the white lines of the ceiling. My face creases into a frown.

'But how could I have had active TB for so long? Dr Taylor said I would be dead . . .'

'Well, I've considered that. Think about all the antibiotics you've had over the years. They would have been constantly dampening it down. Tilly you always say: they never get rid of it; they just calm the infection for a bit.'

I nod.

'I need to go home and research this properly. I don't want to leave you on your own, though. How about we get Finn to come to sit with you?'

I shake my head. I'm not ready to see Finn yet.

She thinks for a moment.

'OK, what about Heidi and Nina? They keep offering to visit. They could come this afternoon and then Dad will be here this evening, after work. Can I message them?'

I met Nina at nursery and we quickly became inseparable. Nina's parents, Heidi and Simon, became my second family, their house my second home. Heidi is Norwegian and as a child I became a regular at their summer house in Norway; holidays of uninterrupted freedom spent adventuring over rugged, wild coastlines.

'OK, but you haven't told them about the TB, have you?'

'I promise you, I haven't.'

'What if someone mentions it?'

'I really don't think Dr Taylor's going to be returning today, after that scene, do you?'

I shake my head.

'What will we say to them?'

'I'll say you've got another nasty infection. You know people don't ask the details and Heidi's not medical. Anyway, you could escape the ward for a bit. Maybe they could take you on a big day out to the hospital cafe?'

I smile.

'Whatever happens while I'm gone, though, you must not take *any* TB drugs.'

While Mum heads down to the hospital entrance to meet Heidi and Nina, I have some rare time alone. I'm craving a moment of quiet to mentally process the events of the last few weeks. It feels like playing back a film in which I'm the main character. It's hard to believe it's happening to me. It winds me deep in my stomach and leaves me gasping for breath. Could something as innocent as a jug of milk on my breakfast cereal have caused all of this?

My thoughts are interrupted by the sound of Mum leading Heidi and Nina into my room.

'Oh, Tilly, we were so worried about you.' Heidi envelops me in a hug. 'And you must be exhausted.' She leans over and puts her arm around Mum's shoulder.

'I'm fine, I'm fine,' Mum smiles.

Before she leaves, Mum begins to hunt for a wheelchair for my great escape to the hospital cafe. After scouring every inch of the ward, it turns out they're in short supply and eventually a nurse has to call a porter on my behalf. Think of it like a hotel concierge service but with an element of suspense: will your transport appear now or in three hours? Nobody knows.

Half an hour later, Ramesh, the porter, arrives in my room.

'Voila,' he grins. 'I found this one hidden in the broom cupboard on the gastro ward.'

We all celebrate its arrival, as if Ramesh has just entered with a Ferrari and not a battered wheelchair with a ripped seat revealing a crumbling foam base.

'Gastro always try to hide them because cardiology keep stealing theirs when no one is looking,' says Ramesh. 'But I've learned the hiding places.' He grins.

It's a cut-throat ward-to-ward battle. You snooze you lose.

'You sound like a good guy to know,' Mum says.

'Now, do you need me to take her?' he asks.

'No thank you, we're all good. You're super busy. We can take Tilly down.'

My legs are wobbly after so many weeks in bed. Mum helps me to manoeuvre onto the chair and then we begin the rickety journey through the corridors. It always feels a little odd emerging from the ward for the first time. I've started to forget there's a whole life out here, beyond my room.

The broken chair screeches and jolts as the brakes crunch along the floor. We emerge in a corridor bathed in the glow of winter sun. Mum pauses and points towards the artwork local schoolchildren have made to adorn the walls. I look up and feel the sun melt into my face. It's lovely to feel its warmth on my skin again. I can't exactly say that we're going to be seeing many of these pieces in the National Gallery any time soon (although you never know – the potato dressed in a floral suit swimming in a sea of psychedelic crabs is quite inspired), but the art lifts my mood, gets us talking about something outside of the medical world and breaks up the endless sterile walls. The children have done a good deed.

We enter the lift, crammed full of patients, visitors and staff with metal trolleys. I try not to breathe, imagining the germs hovering in the stale, claustrophobic air. The lift crunches each time it reaches a new floor. Queues of people wait to get in. Everyone is silent. Everyone is focused on their destination.

As we get out on the ground floor, staff race past us in fast succession. It's hard to identify exactly who's who; they all wear scrubs and they're all in a rush. By contrast, the patients are just waiting. We're all waiting for something – a diagnosis, the right treatment, a visitor, mostly to get better and be discharged home.

En route, we pass overflowing clinics with disparate people spilling out of waiting rooms and down corridors. No one has a connection to each other. No one wants to be here. There are so many crowds of unanchored bodies, brought together only by a quest to be well.

The single-file queue from phlebotomy is metres long. A man at the back is visibly struggling to stand but there are no seats. As we pass, my eyes catch the number on his 'blood ticket': 91. The electronic sign hanging from the ceiling is currently on number 55. I read the poster on the wall behind him:

25p off in Desert Spring Cafe if you show your blood test ticket!

I'm sure a bargain cappuccino will bring a lot of comfort to him during this difficult time.

We move towards the pharmacy, where there are so many people filling the aisles it would be easy to think there was a big Black Friday event taking place. The shoppers are emptying the shelves, jostling to reach the most desirable goods and queuing for as long as it takes to get their hands on the latest products.

The next corridor we enter is lined with bright-orange traffic cones.

'Hospital corridor or roadworks?' I grin.

'I think it's this we should be more worried about.' Heidi points to the ceiling.

I look up and realise that when they say on the news that our poor healthcare system is 'coming apart at the seams' they do actually mean it. The ceiling is being held together by masking tape.

We surge (more like skid) through this particularly dingy – and potentially life-threatening – corridor. Heidi and Nina prove to be very handy assistants, holding open all the heavy double doors, and finally we reach our destination: Desert Spring Cafe.

A trip to the cafe is a chance to escape and yet what I have escaped to is a mix between a prison and a school canteen. The planners clearly forgot to incorporate windows into their design. They did nail the name, though. Desert Spring Cafe offers hot chocolate, tea and coffee – and every single drink tastes like water.

After waving goodbye to Mum, we tuck into our truly

unappetising and dilute drinks, paired with dry-looking cookies. I am not complaining. This is the most excitement I've had in weeks. I look around the cafe and surmise the other patients must feel the same. In one way, it is as depressing as it gets; but in another, it has an energy like nowhere else in the hospital. Everyone in here is free from the wards and savouring every second. Patients congregate from all different parts of the hospital. Next to one man is an oxygen cylinder; another young girl sits with her mum, who's drinking a coffee. The girl has nothing in front of her. I take in her face and realise she's connected to a feeding tube. I stare down at my cookie and feel bad for even thinking it's dry. Another lady wears a bright-pink fluffy dressing gown. She's talking and laughing on the phone. She looks gaunt but happy. Then I catch sight of her legs, poking out from a pair of fleece slippers. I inhale, shocked. People often say 'thin as a twig' but I've never seen anyone *this* thin. Mixed into the scene are doctors and nurses. Some are huddled in groups involved in intense debates, others are shoving in a quick sandwich and snatching a few minutes' catchup with their colleagues. They work tirelessly on the wards night and day and *this* is their oasis.

Desert spring: a thriving source of life in a barren landscape.

Second part, spot on. First part, not so much.

After taking it all in, I do what you have to do to keep going: I block out the scene. I try to imagine I'm out with Heidi and Nina at the weekend and we're having a catchup over coffee (and just in error picked somewhere with a one-star hygiene rating).

'So, how are you *really*?' Heidi asks. She looks directly at me and gently rubs my shoulder. I want to open up. I want to tell her everything but I can't. It feels too scary. What if Heidi tells Simon, then he tells just one other person? That's how these things spread.

'It's not the dream but just the usual,' I smile.

'I guess you're used to it now,' Nina says.

I think back to when Nina and I were at primary school. One day, our headmaster came into assembly to inform us that one of the pupils, Lottie Green, was seriously ill.

'Lottie Green is very poorly. Lottie Green has cancer,' he announced.

When she first ended up in hospital, the school gates were a frenzy of, 'It's a parent's worst nightmare', 'Imagine that happening to our little Johnny' and 'Poor Lottie Green'. Lottie's bedroom was overflowing with cards, toys, sweets and balloons. Within a few weeks, the balloons burst. They were never replaced.

When 'little Johnny' ended up in hospital with a sprained wrist, his parents' whole world stopped. But Lottie Green practically living there? That was *so much better*. It was her second home now. She was *used to it*.

When I first ended up in hospital, all those years ago, the whole class made me a 'get well soon' card, but, like Lottie Green, I wasn't getting better any time soon.

I want to tell Nina she's got it all wrong, that patient life doesn't get easier over time. Not only am I going through the trauma on repeat, but on every admission I know what to expect. My fears are raw and visceral; I anticipate the pain before it happens. Each time I come in, I witness more tragic stories unfold – stories that will stay with me for life. My heart takes just as much of a battering as my body but no one sees these invisible scars, the ones that linger deep within.

I find I can't bring myself to voice the words. It feels safer to let Nina believe that I'm the expert patient, managing just fine, protected by years of experience.

'I couldn't do it,' she says, looking down at the cannula poking out of my bruised arm.

'You could,' I say, 'if you had to.'

The lady at the next table starts to cough, a thick, crackling cough. She grabs a paper towel to press against her face.

'How about we get out of here?' Nina poses.

'Escape?' I grin.

'We could wheel you out to the main entrance for a breath of fresh air. It's cold but it's a beautiful day,' Heidi says.

I agree immediately. Fresh air sounds like the dream. Heidi tucks my blanket around my thighs and wraps me up in her thick puffer jacket. Nina pulls the hood over my head.

'Our little caterpillar,' she laughs.

'I feel a bit like a caterpillar cooped up in here.'

As the cold air hits my face, I lift it up towards the sun and relish the rays soaking into my skin. I savour the feeling of the fresh air biting my cheeks. We all pause for a moment, eyes closed, heads up in the air, smiles on our faces.

'Look!' Heidi points towards the ground.

I steer my eyes away from the blue sky and look down. Growing from a crack in the pavement is a single, bright-yellow dandelion.

'You're a dandelion child, Tilly,' she says.

'What do you mean?' I look up at her, puzzled.

'In Norway we use this phrase to describe children who have grown up in tough circumstances but thrive despite them.'

'Because dandelions bloom anywhere, not just in lush green fields but also in the cracks between the pavement,' Nina adds.

I look down and take in the resilient green stalk and tiny yellow petals flourishing among the rough stones and dirty cigarette butts. I like the idea that I'm a dandelion, upright and strong, with everything crumbling around me.

'I'll never look at dandelions in the same way again.'

The next morning, I am discharged. I'm not sure if this is because I am strictly well enough to leave or if Dr Taylor just wants me out of his hospital. I am handed three months' worth of latent TB drugs, which I am under strict instruction from Mum *not* to take.

Before we leave, there is just one thing we have to do. Today, like clockwork, there are three light taps on my door. Mrs Sarma bobs her head around, with that familiar steaming cup of tea. Mum delves into her bag, then walks towards the door. She hands Mrs Sarma a little box, tied with a white ribbon.

'For you.'

Mrs Sarma bats the gift away.

'No please,' Mum says, 'you must take it. You will never know what you have done for us this week.'

Now Mrs Sarma begins to tear up.

'I told you,' says Mum. 'I really can do anything, as long as I have a cup of tea.'

*

Mum remains certain she's read that this QuantiFERON Gold test *does* test for TB from milk. Knowing the doctors have already discharged me with a prescription for latent treatment, she realises she needs to act quickly. Tonight, she once again stays up until the early hours trawling the internet. Her detective work uncovers an email address for the test manufacturer in America. She sends them a concise email explaining our predicament and asks one key question:

> Does QuantiFERON Gold test for active bovine tuberculosis from milk?

By 5am, the test manufacturer in America has already replied, saying they have forwarded her email to their laboratory in Germany.

Two hours later, another email lands in her inbox. Hagen, the scientist from the lab in Germany, has responded. He confirms that, yes, Mum is right: QuantiFERON Gold *does* test for active bovine TB from unpasteurised milk.

> Under no circumstance must you let your daughter take those latent TB drugs. I have forwarded your email to Dr Ralph, a leading expert on TB in the UK. I urge you to seek his medical opinion.

'TB is known as "the great masquerader",' Dr Ralph tells us at my first appointment, a week later. 'It doesn't want to be caught. Instead, it aims to hide in the body and multiply, causing absolute havoc and, eventually, tries to kill you.'

For 12 years, the TB has been playing a crafty game of hide and seek, concealing its true self and mimicking other illnesses. It's been parading under the glistening lights of the chandelier, an unwelcome guest at a masked ball, unidentifiable in its seamless disguise.

'It's one of the few illnesses that can affect every part of the body, bar the hair on your head,' Dr Ralph informs us.

I always felt I couldn't have this many separate things wrong with me. I was certain there must be one condition that explained them all.

'Could Tilly have had it for so many years?' Mum asks.

'The typical cases most doctors think of these days are someone catching a raging lung infection and instantly being hit with acute symptoms, but TB can present in so many ways. Chronic TB is much more common from drinking unpasteurised milk. It's concealed in the intestine – this is why yours has never been infectious.'

All the clues are now starting to add up.

'You said you study English?' Dr Ralph adds.

I nod.

'Well, think of some of the great poets, Tilly. Before there was a cure, many of them lived with TB for years. They were sent to sanatoriums, to breathe in the fresh air, absorb vitamin D from the sun and conserve their energy.'

I look over at Mum and smile. We've created our own sanatorium. I realised long ago that any form of exertion equalled infection. So, for years, I've barely moved. I've always craved the sunshine, basking in it at every opportunity. It feels particularly poignant that

I'm studying the Romantic poets this term. I think of Keats's ode 'To Autumn', written in the early stages of his tuberculosis.

> Steady thy laden head across a brook;
> Or by a cyder-press, with patient look,
> Thou watchest the last oozings hours by hours.

Keats's rich, lyrical imagery on the themes of patience and fulfilment feel so relevant to my own life at this very moment. Today, Dr Ralph hands me a prescription for active bovine tuberculosis. With that, my fears about the future begin to fall away like the mellow fruits and autumn leaves. A new season, ripe with possibility, awaits.

It takes me a while to pluck up the courage to own my label. I agonise for weeks about telling Finn. I'm not sure what I am scared of exactly; I guess being seen as anything other than 'Tilly'. My way of coping has always been to compartmentalise my life, but over time I realise that my relationship can never flourish with this huge secret at its centre. I have to let Finn in. I lie next to him on his bed and whisper those three words:

'I have tuberculosis.'

It's as if by saying them quietly, they'll appear less shocking – less real somehow. Finn stares up at the ceiling, quiet for a moment. I hold my breath, waiting for him to respond. Then he turns towards me, places his hands around mine and looks directly into my eyes.

'Tilly, from now on, this is something we deal with *together*.'

For so long I've been out at sea, my head gently bobbing above the surface, concealing my legs frantically treading water below. Finn's words are like a life ring. I now have something to hold onto, someone else to share this momentous burden with. I no longer need to use every grain of energy to keep up my façade.

We stay up talking most of the night. I recount the whole story: Aunt Nora's farm, the milk, the cow that ruined my life. However shocked he may be feeling on the inside, he remains outwardly steadfastly calm.

'I'm not going anywhere,' he repeats.

Finn is there to help me stay afloat and, for now, that is enough.

I'm still certain that if everyone at university finds out, I will simply be referred to as 'that girl in fourth year, you know the one with TB'. So, Finn is under strict instruction not to tell anyone. For the duration of my treatment, I tell my friends I have a 'rare bacteria' and leave it at that. No one pushes me for answers. It is only after we graduate that I give my illness a name. Once I'm out of the university bubble, it somehow doesn't seem as big. With each person I tell, it's like a new lifebuoy is thrown out to me at sea. I'm no longer spending my life furiously kicking behind the scenes.

Eighteen months on, when I finish my treatment, I'm floating through life, held up by all the people I've finally let in.

PATIENT SURVIVAL TIPS

- Try sharing this scenario to those around you: think about being stabbed with a needle once (*ouch*). Now think about being stabbed with a needle one hundred times. Pose the question: what's worse?
- For patients and loved ones, if the opportunity to step outside of the ward for just a few minutes arises, seize it. Some gulps of fresh air, a vending-machine chocolate bar and a (lukewarm) coffee will transform you.
- Are you searching for a diagnosis? It's time to put on your detective hat; question everything, pursue all avenues and take nothing as fact.
- You are *not* the crack in the pavement. You are *not* your illness. You *are* the dandelion.
- When life feels futile, sometimes it takes just one person to restore our faith in humanity.

Part 2
CRISIS

10

GAPS

For so long, I've been a sunflower desperately trying to bloom, but trapped in a stained vase filled with gungy water and left without light. The TB treatment makes me golden again. There's no dramatic moment, more a gradual return to sunnier days and clearer waters. I'm finally aware of what it is to feel healthy again. The paradox of this is that the stronger I grow, the more *unaware* I become. To start with, minutes go by where I'm not actively thinking about my body causing havoc, then hours, then days and even weeks pass. The mental space this opens is liberating. No longer is every second of the day devoted to navigating my symptoms.

For the first year of treatment, there are, of course, still moments where my brain jumps back into fear mode. After being ill for this long, this has become an automatic reflex. A slight cough or a twinge in my lung and I instantly fast forward to a future of pneumonias, hospitals and IV antibiotics. Two years on, though, there are no pneumonias and I start to allow myself to believe that this is really it.

During these golden years, I begin to live the sort of 'ordinary' life I've always dreamed about. I reclaim all the time that used to be spent travelling to hospitals, sitting in waiting rooms, attending appointments and organising the endless admin of patient life. I no longer live out my days on the sofa. I begin to exercise; a bit of gentle yoga to start with and then a short walk. I don't just nibble at tiny portions of food but notice that I'm actually *hungry*. To start with, this feeling is so alien I question it. Then I realise that this is what 'healthy' people must feel multiple times a day. This basic human instinct is a sign that my body is *working*.

When, six months after finishing my treatment, Finn suggests we move into a flat in London together, the timing feels just right. In the past, I had to rely on my parents to drive me places, arrange prescriptions, join me at medical appointments, pick up my shopping and cook me food, and that's not to mention all the emotional support they gave me too. I know when you love someone you *want* to do these things, but being on the receiving end always made me so aware of how different my life was from other people's. I yearned to be standing at my own hob, making my own pasta, shrinking my own cotton T-shirt or deciding what to put in my own shopping basket. For so many years, this illness robbed me of my independence. Moving away from home now feels like a momentous step.

After graduation, Finn and most of my friends had started working in London. I was still on my TB treatment and wasn't in a position to work full time. I was so worried future employers were going to notice the huge gap on my CV. It was then that I hit on the idea of launching my own student platform. Although I'd dreamed of going to Oxford Uni, I found the whole process of applying terrifying, especially given how much school I'd missed. So, after graduating, I decided to set up (from my bed) a free resource to help other applicants overcome barriers. This gave me the flexibility to work on my own terms, while I was recovering, and became my 'something good out of something bad'.

The only problem now is that it doesn't really pay the bills. To be able to move to London with Finn and contribute to our extortionate rent, I quickly need to find a paid job.

'We've taken a look through your CV,' Lewis, the director of the recruitment company, says at the beginning of my interview. 'I notice there's been quite a gap over the last year.'

My heart drops. This is the question I feared he would ask, the question I have agonised over for months.

'Well, Lewis, I actually took most of the year out to . . . lie on the sofa.'

That's not going to cut it. I'm certain that if I share my actual story with Lewis, he won't want to take the risk on me. 'The Girl with TB' continues to haunt me.

'I came up with the concept for the student platform I recently launched, and spent time planning that,' I smile.

'Mm, yes, I understand that's why you are looking for more of a freelance, part-time role with us.'

I nod.

'Did you do anything else, though? It's been over a year since you graduated . . .'

'Erm, yes, I went travelling.'

'Oh, how wonderful, where?'

Time to make my weekend mini-break to Malaga sound like a cultural tour of Europe.

'I visited Spain for a while. I have a keen interest in taking up Spanish in my spare time.'

I really hope Lewis isn't fluent in Spanish.

He grills me for a while longer. Then he asks me to remain seated while he heads out of the room for a moment. I take a few deep breaths and a couple of sips of water.

Minutes later, Lewis pokes his head around the door and guides me into the office next door. I'm faced with a semicircle of what I assume are employees all standing up and grinning at me expectantly.

Lewis turns to me.

'Tilly, we would like to offer you the job.'

The other people all start clapping.

'Oh, wow, erm . . . great, thank you!' I smile.

Lewis leans over to shake my hand. The way they are all acting, I feel like I've just been offered shares in a multimillion-pound business. Alas, that's not the case. Instead, I am officially a freelance, part-time recruiter. Dreams really do come true. I can now move into a flat so small it's effectively a cupboard, but I could not be happier. For the first time in forever, I am going to be independent.

For six months, life remains golden. I'm blissfully ensconced with Finn, in our tiny flat kitted out with Ikea flatpack furniture. We work hard and play hard, throwing ourselves into London life: cocktails after work, brunches in over-hyped cafes with no booking policies and Sunday afternoons whiled away in pub gardens. We grab morning coffees together en route to the tube and when we get back from work, we share everything about our day over bowls of pesto pasta.

'Urgh, I had another nightmare today,' I say to Finn, as we curl up on the sofa tonight.

My student platform is continuing to grow. I've now set up brand deals with businesses and even launched a team of student ambassadors. Messages from applicants saying how much it has helped on their university journeys always give me such a warm, fuzzy feeling. Sadly, this passion does not extend to recruitment. Lewis has, for some reason, made me solely focus on recruiting coders. I now spend my days bombarding extremely clever tech experts with messages and invites to meet me in posh London hotels.

'The guy told me he used Python and I genuinely thought he was referring to his pet snake.'

Finn looks at me blankly.

'Apparently Python is a coding language.'

We both lie back on the sofa with our hands over our faces and laugh. I take in that magnetic glint in Finn's eye. I want to savour this moment forever. To most people, I'm sure tonight would just be an ordinary evening, but to me there is something brilliant about being ordinary. For years, I had so many critical, lifechanging things to worry about that everything else became irrelevant. I used to dream of having the brain space to worry about something insignificant, something that didn't really matter. I knew when that day came, it would mean life was better.

Now, I am moaning about a mortifying encounter with a recruitment candidate who, in all likelihood, I'll never see again. That day is finally here.

Tonight, I head over to one of my best friends, Liv's flat for girls' night. We met aged two, at a toddler music class, and I will forever be grateful we chose to hit the same tambourine, leading our mums to meet across the crowded room. Liv's a fiery redhead in every sense: bold, loud, hilarious and always the top hostess. The evening starts off pretty great. My home girls Pheobe, Sammi and Eve are all in attendance and Liv has spent hours honing the perfect chilli margaritas. After a few hours of sipping on cocktails and catching up at Liv's, we Uber to a new bar that's just opened in North London. For the first half of the journey, I'm lapping up Sammi's story about her colleague who recently quit his job to run a silent retreat in Thailand.

'He literally only speaks once a month. Can you imagine?'

'I can't imagine *you* doing it, no!' I laugh.

In front of me, the lights of the London skyline start dancing. They merge together in colourful, wavy lines. I wind down the window and take a few breaths.

'You OK, Tilly?' Phoebe asks.

'Yeah, yeah, just a bit hot.'

My head feels a bit fuzzy. A film of sweat seeps across my forehead. I stick my face out of the window, embracing the icy January air. Sammi turns around from the front seat and begins swiping through a montage of her ex-colleague in various yoga poses on a white sandy beach. I try to focus but the photos are all blurry. I can make out the outlines but none of the detail. How much have I had to drink? I think back. I had the one margarita in the kitchen and then I only had a few sips of a second one before we left.

The Uber slows.

'Thanks,' I murmur, stepping outside. My legs feel shaky. I look down at my heels. That will be why.

We gather in the queue, all laughing and gabbling away. The scene is happening around me, but I feel separate. Eve flings her arm on my shoulder. I copy her motion.

Inside, we head over to the bar to order drinks. A few sips in, my heart starts pounding in my chest. I try to ignore it, bobbing for a while, feigning laughter, a smile stamped on my face. Then, suddenly, I can't smile anymore. I'm going to be sick. I make to run in the direction of the toilets but my legs won't carry me. They begin to buckle. I feel an arm around me. What's happening?

When I open my eyes, I'm sitting on the floor of a grimy toilet cubicle. Phoebe is next to me, her hand clasping my shoulder.

'Tilly, Tilly, are you OK? Tilly, how much did you drink?'

I know what I want to say. I want to say, 'I drank one marg before we left, some sips of a second one, and a few sips of wine here,' but that isn't what comes out. What comes out is a jumble of slurred words that make no sense.

Phoebe holds my head in her hands.

'Tilly, what's going on?'

A sharp pain sears deep in my right eyebrow. My head feels like it's going to explode. I press my hands into my scalp. Within seconds I'm in a ball, screaming. My screams pierce through the bassy music. They fly across the cubicles. I can't stop.

'Tilly, Tilly, what's wrong?'

The pain floods my head from top to bottom, drowning my brain. My screams get louder.

'Hey, hey,' a voice calls from outside the cubicle. 'Get your drunk friend out of here!'

'Tilly, Tilly, we need to move you,' Pheobe says.

'NO! NO!' I cry. I can't move. I can't do anything but focus on the pain. It's now ricocheting through my flank.

'Tilly, I'm scared. I need to get some help. I haven't got any signal in here.'

'I'm going to call the bouncers!' the voice shouts from outside.

'Tilly, I'm so sorry, we need to move.'

I crouch in a ball, gripping my head, swaying from side to side.

'BOUNCER INCOMING!' a male voice shouts.

Phoebe stands up and eases open the cubicle door.

'Stand up!' a man shouts.

'Stop being so rude,' I hear Phoebe say. 'She's not drunk. She's really unwell.'

'Yeah, yeah, heard that one before.'

'Tilly, we need to get you out. I think we need to go to hospital.'

Hospital? Did she say hospital? I try to stand but my legs won't hold me up. I wobble and then fall to the floor. I can't work out how it happens, but suddenly I'm being carried past a crowd of people. Phoebe is on one side of me and a man is on the other. My arms are around their shoulders, my legs hanging limply beneath.

'It's OK, Tilly,' Phoebe says.

A heavy set of doors swing open. The cold air hits me. I am back on the ground, shivering.

'I'm just calling the girls. We're going to get you some help, Tilly. Give me two mins.'

Phoebe realises something is seriously wrong and, after grabbing Sammi, Liv and Eve to help her, Ubers me straight to hospital. The driver has to stop multiple times for me to throw up by the kerb. That's our five-star rating down the drain. As our group of five girls in heels and cocktail dresses descend on A&E, I am initially treated as a drunk.

'She has a really complicated medical history. She's not been off TB treatment for long. Please run some tests,' Phoebe pleads with them.

The A&E doctor is having none of it. I am attached to a fluid drip and left. The others are asked to remain in the waiting room but Phoebe is allowed to sit in the chair beside me. She calls Finn, who immediately jumps from bed and heads to the hospital. At 3am, he eventually persuades a reluctant Sammi, Liv and Eve to head home. For the rest of the night, Finn and Phoebe never leave my side.

Eight hours later, my body is still shaking. A doctor bobs his head around my curtain.

'How's she doing this morning?' he asks.

'Something's not right. Look, she's still shaking,' Finn says.

'It will take a bit of time for the alcohol to get out of her system.'

'I keep telling you all, this isn't alcohol,' says Phoebe. 'She had no more to drink than the rest of us.'

I turn to look at Phoebe. Her lace-trimmed, hot-pink slip dress is certainly adding a touch of glamour to A&E but it's not really helping my cause. She may as well be holding up a sign saying 'BIG NIGHT OUT'.

'Can you not take some bloods?' Finn asks.

'No point. She just needs to keep drinking lots of water and she'll feel better.'

Phoebe leans forward in her chair.

'She was in agony, though, screaming with head pain and back pain. Would alcohol do that?'

'We all know what a bad hangover feels like,' the doctor smiles.

This is so not a hangover.

'She's good to go whenever you want to take her.' He turns to talk to me now. 'We advise you go home, drink lots of water and get some rest.'

Finn looks concerned.

'I'm not sure we should go yet, Tilly.'

My whole body is quivering, I feel horrendous but the pain has settled down and I think I'll be able to walk now. I can see we're getting absolutely nowhere here. They've all made up their minds that I was just drunk. They aren't looking for anything else.

'I want to get out of here,' I whisper.

We sit in silence on the way home, staring out at the miserable dawn sky. I glance down at my phone and notice the date.

'Shit, shit – Finn and I are meant to be driving up north with my parents today for my nephew's christening.'

'That's not going to happen, Tilly,' Phoebe says.

I shake my head. I'm meant to be godmother.

'*Unfortunately, your aunt couldn't be here today because she got smashed last night . . .*' I cover my hands over my face. This is not ideal for any family event.

'Maybe by the time he's 18, my nephew will think I'm a bit of a legend.'

They both laugh, but worry is still etched across their faces.

'Do you think your drink was spiked?' Phoebe asks.

'I can't work it out. I'm sure I felt funny before and I only had a few sips of wine at the bar.'

'It just seemed so sudden. You were in so much pain. It was really scary.'

'I'm so sorry, Phoebe. I ruined your night. I ruined everyone's night. I'm so embarrassed.'

'You have absolutely nothing to be embarrassed about, Tilly. We were just worried about you.'

We pull up outside Phoebe's flat. I can't muster the energy to get out of the car to give her the proper hug she deserves but I do lean over and squeeze her hand.

'You really are such a good friend. Thank you.'

As soon as we get back to ours, Finn tucks me up in bed with a hot-water bottle.

'Thank you for coming last night,' I say.

He kisses me lightly on the forehead.

'I feel so bad I ruined everyone's night.'

'No one thinks that. Stop worrying and get some sleep.'

I wake a few hours later and am hit by a sudden wave of nausea. I make it to the bathroom, where I lie against the cool tiled floor in between rounds of more violent vomiting. My only comfort is being grounded. As soon as I rise from the floor, it hits me again.

'I think we need to get you checked out properly,' Finn says.

He calls the GP surgery, where there are, of course, no appointments.

'Ask them to speak to Dr Murphy,' I whisper.

Years ago, when Dr Murphy realised I was the ultimate 'zebra', he put a note on my file, asking to be alerted if I ever called requesting an urgent appointment.

A few minutes later, the receptionist calls back.

'Dr Murphy's said to come in immediately,' Finn says.

This was the exact reason why, when I moved to London, I decided to stay registered with my GP surgery back home. They're only 30 minutes away and this kind of continuity of care offered by a doctor who actually knows me is gold dust.

By the time we arrive at the surgery, my legs have once again turned feathery and won't hold me up. Finn runs to get a wheelchair and pushes me into the waiting room. This is some hangover.

Unlike the doctors in A&E, Dr Murphy knows my weird and wonderful medical history and actually runs some blood tests.

'It's probably a bit late now, as you've been on fluids, but we'll check just in case.'

Next, he takes my blood sugar.

'It's very low, Tilly.'

'What does that mean?'

'I'm not sure,' he acknowledges. 'Is it possible your drink was spiked?'

I shrug. It doesn't quite ring true with me but I can't think of another explanation.

PATIENT SURVIVAL TIPS

- Any small achievement while being unwell is a strength, not a weakness that you have to hide.
- If the universe gives you a break, don't cloud it with worry about tomorrow. Embrace today.
- Patient life can rob you of your independence. Find one little thing per day that you can do on your own to regain control.
- Your friends love you for *you*.
- Continuity of care can be game-changing; request to see a GP who knows you.

11

WILTING

It happens so gradually that to start with, I tell myself I'm imagining it. I so want to be in my golden era, I convince myself that is where I remain; but slowly my smooth, golden petals become frayed at the tips and, over time, the very core of me begins to wilt. Ever since the possible 'spiked drink' incident, something hasn't been right. The bloods all came back normal but for three days afterwards, my whole body continued to shake. In the months since, I've developed a list of nondescript symptoms: leg cramps, flank pain, morning nausea, dizziness and exhaustion. The only pattern I can find is that I always feel better as the day goes on. I'm terrified to admit to myself that I'm feeling poorly again, let alone to Finn. We've done the 'illness' bit, ticked it off. This is meant to be the new, 'normal' phase of our relationship. In my attempts to hide it, I've found I'm back to doing two things I thought I had firmly put behind me: pretending and adapting. My job means my hours are quite flexible and I can often work from home. During the week, by the time Finn returns to our flat, my body has often kicked back into action enough to function. Weekends are harder.

'Is everything OK?' Finn asks, as my eyes flicker open.

I roll over and tap my phone. My flank stabs. I try not to wince. It's almost 1pm. We didn't even go out last night. I opted for a 'chilled Saturday' again, on the pretence that I'd had a super-busy week. I tilt my head up to look at Finn. His eyes remain glued to his tablet. I know his question is loaded. What he's really saying is: are *we* OK? I've barely seen him over the last few weeks. It's so much harder to pretend when we're both together and I just haven't had the energy. Rather than having to face him, I've made excuses, told him I have plans with the girls and feigned many a stressful day at work.

'Just needed to catch up on sleep,' I say. Not exactly a lie.

He scans my face. I can almost see the thoughts toying in his brain as he contemplates whether to push this any further. In the end, he returns to his tablet.

'I'll go shower,' I murmur.

I drag myself to the bathroom and analyse my reflection in the mirror. I actually look pretty well. I almost have a glow about me, but it doesn't match how I feel inside. A wave of nausea takes over and I begin to retch over the toilet. This has become a bit of a pattern now. I don't actually throw up, just find myself repeatedly dry heaving. It's grim. Once the sickness calms a bit, I clean my teeth and have a cold shower.

'We need to head soon for Luke's lunch,' Finn says, when I return to the bedroom.

Urgh, I forgot it was Luke's birthday. I can't face sitting at a table all afternoon. I want to go back to bed.

'I might have to give it a miss,' I say. 'I have a load of work to catch up on.'

'You can't work all the time, Tilly. Luke's one of your best mates.'

'I don't work all the time. I've just had a busy week.'

'You always seem to be busy at the moment.'

'Why are you being funny?' I snap.

'I'm not. You're the one being funny. You're either busy, asleep or, when we're together, you seem kind of off.'

Finn's right but I can't explain it. I can't explain any of it. I know I'm withdrawing, wrapping that protective guard around myself and pushing him away. It feels easier to hide than to face up to feeling ill again.

'Sorry, I've just had a stressful few weeks.' I lean over to kiss him. 'Of course I'll come.'

So, I do what I have done for so long: I pretend. I physically haul myself onto the tube. My weak legs somehow carry me to the pub and I sit at the table, talking, laughing and picking at food I can't stomach. All the while, I assume a carefree smile. To the outside world, life looks good.

The only person I properly talk to about all of this is Mum.

'You can't go on like this, Tilly. Try to book an appointment with Dr Murphy and explain to him what's happening. I'm sure he'll try to help you,' she says, after weeks observing me going downhill.

It takes me a while to pluck up the courage to make the appointment – it's as if taking myself back to the doctor's surgery means I'll have to admit the very truth I don't want to face: I'm ill. I want to believe I'm just a bit run down or I've just caught a little bug, but I know that's not true. I know what it is to be *really* ill and

I know this isn't going away on its own. Sometimes things get so bad, they become impossible to ignore.

Two weeks later, I'm back in the waiting room.

'Dr Murphy's off sick today, so you will be seeing Dr Chandra,' the receptionist says.

'No problem,' I smile. This is actually a huge problem. Dr Murphy knows me and he knows I only ever book an appointment when there is something seriously wrong. Trying to explain my bizarre medical history to someone new always takes up the entire slot, leaving little room to discuss anything else. I've waited over two weeks for this appointment, though, so there's no turning back.

It goes just as predicted.

'I think this is probably down to anxiety,' Dr Chandra says. 'These are all classic signs of panic attacks and the body responding to stress.'

I think of all the stress I've had to deal with over the years. It's never made me throw up or scream in pain.

'I know where you're coming from,' I begin. 'But in the past I was told by several doctors that stress was the cause of my symptoms and it turned out I had TB. I do feel these are *physical* symptoms, not connected to any particularly stressful situation.'

I teeter along that fine line of trying to get my point across without sounding in any way like the 'expert patient'.

'Stress can manifest in all sorts of physical ways,' Dr Chandra says.

'I just find it a little hard to imagine I'm so stressed while I'm asleep. Sometimes the pain wakes me.'

Those must be some stressful dreams.

'You couldn't be pregnant?' she poses.

'Nope.'

'You said life has been quite busy since you moved to London.'

I slowly nod.

'I think it's probably just too much to cope with after your past trauma. It's something that may be helpful to talk through with someone.'

My 'past trauma' is well and truly in the *past* and I could not be happier. My only trauma right now is feeling too unwell to focus on *present* fun.

'Are you open to counselling?'

I know how this works. If I say no, I'll look like I won't accept help. If I say yes, I'll have to devote another part of my week to therapy, and time is something I'm already struggling to manage as it is. It's going to take up energy I just don't have.

'Of course. If you think it will help,' I smile brightly.

She nods and begins filling out a form.

'While I am happy to go to counselling, I do feel quite a lot of these symptoms are very physical,' I say again. 'Could you possibly do any bloods or refer me to anyone for more tests?'

'One thing at a time. Otherwise, we won't know what's helping, will we?'

I know I have to play the game.

Mid-writing, she glances up.

'Oh, and you may not have noticed: your dungarees.'

I look down at my trademark black jersey dungarees. They are inside-out. After dragging myself from my bed and heading to the toilet for my ritualistic retch, I threw them on, without even looking, to race out of the door in time for this appointment.

I can already see the note on my counselling referral: *Tilly has reached the stage where her mental capacity for day-to-day tasks, like dressing herself, is now being affected.*

Life is now seriously beginning to spiral. I've started setting an alarm for midday and then attempting to get most of my work done from my bed. I'm popping paracetamol every four hours for pain. I'm having regular cold showers to blast myself awake. I'm dragging myself outside on short walks around the block. I'm doing everything I can but it's not enough.

I look at healthy people, whose bodies just seem to work on an automatic reflex, and yearn to be like them. Mine seems to require so much conscious thought. Endless days and nights are spent second-guessing, responding and coming up with strategies. The brain space that was previously taken up trying to solve the TB diagnosis has now been filled again, with hours spent trawling the internet for my vague list of symptoms. Terms like 'weakness', 'exhaustion', 'headache' and 'irritability' aren't exactly narrowing my search. It's starting to feel utterly futile. I'm not sure I can keep doing it; I'm exhausted by the very act of trying.

I tell myself that maybe the stress and trauma of having been unwell for so many years is only just starting to show – maybe counselling will be the answer. The logical part of my brain speaks louder, though: these are new, *physical* symptoms and they are getting worse.

'This is ridiculous,' Mum says, when I tell her about Dr Chandra's referral. 'Your symptoms are physical.'

Sometimes it takes someone else to confirm what you already know.

'I can't win,' I say. 'If I turn it down, I get told I'm not helping myself and if I accept, I make it so easy for them to put everything down to stress.'

'I know, Tilly, the system makes no sense. Maybe go along. You never know, it may help to talk, but don't in any way be railroaded into thinking this is all in your head.'

Over the years, Mum and I have always talked everything through. She's so solution-focused, which is just what I like. Whenever I go to her with a problem, she comes up with something new we can try – whether that's emailing a new doctor, asking about a new medication or trying a different supplement. This has allowed me to always feel I'm regaining a little control. Having a plan has become my coping mechanism.

'You know I'll never stop looking,' Mum assures me.

I feel like a spider constructing its web; each day adding more and more threads to the complex design. From the outside, I'm creating a fine, luminous vision of perfection, but it's becoming ever more fragile. The worse I feel, the more prey I'm trapping. Mum is now stuck in my web, unable to escape. I'm so tired of being the spider. I'm so tired of feeling guilty.

'I'm so sorry, Mum. I hate the way this illness isn't just ruining my life but yours too.'

'You must never be sorry, Tilly. This has always been my choice. No one has ever made me do it. I've *chosen* to never let this go.'

I think on it for a moment.

'No, Mum, you never chose this. You do it because you love me.'

She squeezes my hand.

'Love isn't a choice,' I say.

Mum wraps her arm around me.

'You're right, Tilly. Loving you has never been a choice.'

I know that behind the scenes, out of my view, Mum will now devote her days and nights to being a medical detective again. That's the bit that hurts, the 'again'. This phase of her life was meant to be over. I want Mum to be out with her friends, off on holidays with Dad, not crouched over her laptop 24/7, trying to solve another medical mystery. I'll do whatever it takes to set us all free and if that's now counselling, then sign me up.

'Do you wash?' the lady on the end of the phone asks me.

I didn't really envisage this being how I would regain control of my life. My mental-health assessor, Sue, from Dr Chandra's referral, seems intent on discussing my hygiene habits. Washing feels like a real deal-breaker in terms of whether I'll make it through to the coveted next round: an *in-person* counselling session.

'Yes, I do, when I'm feeling well enough.'

'So, you don't *always* wash?'

'Well, no, because some days I now feel too ill to even get out of bed, so even a shower is a huge effort.'

'Right, I have to tick a box, you see. So, I need to know if it's "most days" or "weekly" or "don't wash".'

'Well, on the days I feel well enough to get out of bed, I always wash.'

'Ah I see. Do you often feel too down to actually get out of bed, then?'

'No, not down. I feel too weak.'

'Right, OK, erm . . .' Sue pauses. 'Shall we just tick "some days" you wash?'

Showering, along with a lot of the other 'normal' things in my life, has become a struggle, not because I'm depressed and can't face retreating from beneath my duvet but because my body has become so weak that showering feels like running a marathon. Two very legitimate but *different* reasons for not washing. Sue's form leaves no room for this distinction.

'Have you ever tried to kill yourself?'

This question appears from nowhere. It jolts me.

'Erm, no, no I haven't.'

'Have you ever *thought* about killing yourself?'

'No.'

Sue informs me that because I'm not 'actively suicidal', all she can offer me for now is some support with 'managing my anxiety'.

'That sounds really helpful,' I say, imagining this will involve sitting down and having a chat with a caring counsellor who will help me get rid of the tight knot in my tummy. What it actually involves is a PowerPoint presentation.

After double checking that Finn is definitely out of the flat, I flick through the slides Sue has emailed over. They are titled

'Understanding Anxiety', 'Challenging Thoughts' and 'Managing Worry'.

I stare at the black-and-white presentation on the screen. I'd say it resembles a corporate seminar but that gives it too much credit – Finn's finance presentations are far more engaging than this. I read that 'Anxiety is a normal human response to danger or threat'. The only danger or threat to me right now is everyone believing this is all in my head.

One of the slides has an exercise labelled 'Time', 'Thought' and 'Feeling', the idea being that you note down what thought is in your head at the exact moment you're experiencing the stressful feeling. It informs me that this will be a helpful way to work out what's triggering my anxiety. I trace my eyes over the words and conclude that the problem is that I don't think my thoughts do match my feelings. The anxiety or stress just envelops me at random intervals, like an uncontrollable rush of adrenaline.

The PowerPoint ends by telling me:

Every change you make for the better will have lots of benefits.

It doesn't exactly sound transformative but I'm desperate. I'll take 'lots of benefits' for now. I'll take *anything* that might make me feel better.

PATIENT SURVIVAL TIPS

- Mindset isn't everything when your body doesn't work.
- Share your situation with someone who knows you well and will tell you, honestly, what they think – not just what you want to hear.
- GPs can be the gatekeepers to a host of specialists; if you believe there's a problem, keep returning.
- Celebrate the small wins. Some days simply having a shower is an achievement.
- Even the brightest sunflowers wilt if they aren't tended. If you find yourself fading, ask for help to bloom again.

12

WAVES

For the next few weeks, every time I'm overcome by that anxious tug, I pull out my sheet of paper and note down the time and how I'm feeling. The part that proves more difficult is the 'Thought' bit. One day, I'm listening to an upbeat song on the radio while driving and then – suddenly, mid-lyric – I'm on the verge of tears. Another evening, I'm lying on the sofa with Finn, watching a gripping BBC crime drama we're obsessed with, when as if from nowhere stress floods through me, bringing down my mood in an instant. The third time, I'm reeling off my repetitive copy-and-paste messages to coding candidates when my heart starts racing and the knot in my tummy tightens so much it winds me. I stare down at the boxes and struggle to know what to write. I can't match my thoughts to my feelings. The first time, I'd been thinking what a great song was playing. The next time, I'd been contemplating whether the main character Cheryl was having an affair with her best friend's husband. And the third time, I'd been wondering why Rick from Essex would ever leave the highly successful electric-vehicle startup he founded to apply for a dull coding role in a Bedfordshire accountancy firm. I'm not sure this is what the PowerPoint had in mind.

I spend a lot of time replaying the exercises but I'm just not convinced anxiety is the reason for my growing list of symptoms. This afternoon, I'm mulling it all over while pulling out of a bay in the supermarket car park. My heart starts racing and my head begins to spin. Suddenly my car is shunted forwards. The force of another vehicle penetrates through the back of my seat, jolting my body. I automatically shout out, my hands tightly clasping the wheel to steady myself. I fling my head around to look out of the rear windscreen. I gasp. *Oh no, oh no, what have I done? I've reversed into another car. How? How did I not see it? Why wasn't I looking?*

A man is now climbing out of a beige estate, his arms flung up in the air. He looks annoyed. I mean, fair enough. I'd be annoyed too. I jump out of my seat and do the thing that every insurance company unofficially advises you not to do.

'I am *so* sorry; I am so, so sorry. That was completely my fault. I don't know what happened . . .'

He asks me to manoeuvre to the far end of the car park, where we can chat and check his car. I kind of want to ask if *he* can move my car, given I clearly shouldn't be allowed on the roads.

Thankfully, there's no real damage. He points to a supposed dent that I'm struggling to see. I just go with it, desperate to make my escape. I hand over my number, apologise at least 20 more times, offer to pay for any damage and then immediately call Finn.

'Can you come and get me?' I whisper down the phone.

Finn races down the road to meet me and drives our car home.

When I cross the threshold into our flat, I break down in tears. You tread water for a while, desperately trying to hold it together, and then, finally, one small wave pushes you under. Today, that wave was a beige estate car in the supermarket car park. Now I'm drowning and I don't know how to reach the surface.

'What's going on, Tilly?' Finn asks, catching me heaving over the toilet.

I wipe my sleeve across my mouth and lean back against the bathroom wall, wrapping my arms around my legs and leaning my chin against my knees. I stare ahead and remain silent. I don't know what to say. I don't know what's happening to me. Finn joins me on the floor, placing his hand on my knee.

'You can't keep pretending.'

'My body's been ill for so long. Maybe it's just taking a bit of time to recover,' I murmur.

'No, you were doing so well, but something's changed in the last few months.'

I know Finn's right. I so much want to be jumping into our new life. The willpower is there but it's becoming obvious that my body's holding me back.

'Tell me what's going on.'

I take a breath and begin to talk. I tell him about my strange symptoms. I tell him about the GP. I tell him about the PowerPoint I've studiously committed to. Until now, Finn and I have been living together but really I've been alone, lost in a dark forest, trying to navigate my fears with Mum from afar. Now Finn has joined us in the forest. There isn't yet a clear path out but there is another person by my side to hold me tight, to assure me it will be OK and to help me formulate a plan. I no longer have to hide behind the trees; I can step out into the glade. The forest feels a little less daunting now.

'We'll get through this, just like we did before,' Finn says.

I pause for a moment and look up at him.

'Why do you want to be with me?' I ask. 'You could be with someone healthy; someone who can do all the things you want to do with your life. Instead, you're stuck with me.'

'Because I love you, Tilly.'

'But why? I can't give you the life that you want.'

'The life I want is with *you*.'

I look down at my crumpled body, leaning against the bathroom tiles. Finn should run, escape the forest and leave me behind.

'And what are you going to do, Tilly?'

I know exactly what he wants me to say but I turn my head away.

'How can I "beat it", when we don't even know what "it" is?'

Over the next few weeks, things deteriorate further. I wake every morning with a sharp, stabbing pain in my flank. If I don't set an alarm for midday I sleep right through. Most days, I feel so sick I can't stomach any food until the afternoon. I'm losing weight. My legs are weak and feathery. I'm constantly dizzy. To top it all off, I've also developed this weird blotchy tan line above my top lip, which is starting to look like an unkempt moustache.

Eventually, I decide my web is becoming too heavy; it's hanging by a single thread and in one swift motion could all fall down.

'I think I should go back home to Mum and Dad's this weekend,' I say to Finn.

Within seconds of me walking through the door, Mum realises things have taken a serious turn for the worse. She resumes her role as full-time medical researcher and encourages me to try to book an appointment with Dr Murphy in the meantime.

'Specifically say you need to see him and you don't mind waiting longer. It will be worth it, Tilly. He knows you.'

Two weeks later, Dr Murphy confirms there's a serious problem – though he doesn't know what – and immediately makes a referral. Over the next couple of months, I begin the familiar rounds of medics and tests, a futile loop of doors opening and closing. When the answer isn't immediately obvious, the doctors pass me on. It feels like I'm retracing a past I thought I had firmly left behind.

This morning, I'm lying in bed torturing myself with fears of a future held captive to another unknown illness when Mum enters my room holding a beautiful bunch of flowers.

'From Jess,' she smiles.

Back when we were at uni, the year after Finn and I got 'college married', we were allocated Jess as our 'college daughter' when the new cohort of students arrived. I'd spent most of her first term in hospital, so barely saw her to start with, but we had an instant bond. Ever since then, whenever things have become particularly bad and this illness has forced me to retreat away from life, Jess has always sent me flowers.

I look across at the blast of pink peonies Mum is now arranging in a vase on my bedside table. These little gestures matter so much when you're stuck in the same place day in, day out.

'Peonies are the healing flower,' Mum says to me.

I stare ahead despondently. I'm so far from healed.

Mum joins me on the bed, with her laptop.

'I've come up with a new plan,' she says. 'I think it could be something hormonal. Your body's all over the place and this could affect your emotions as well. What do you think about these?' She points to a list of medical conditions she's organised into a neat bullet-point list.

I tell my mind to remain numb and uninterested, not to engage, but I can't stop myself and a flicker of curiosity sparks from within. Mum knows I love a plan. I peel my eyes away from the wall to face the laptop screen. As I scan the page, hope and fear meet at the edge of a precipice. Fear makes me want to slam the laptop shut and hide away forever cocooned in my duvet. Hope is the reassuring hand, pulling me forward and offering the possibility of a new path.

'Yes, you're right. Any of these could be me,' I say.

'We shouldn't have to do this, Tilly, but I think we might have to book a private endocrinology appointment. Otherwise, it will be months until you're seen. We can't leave you like this.'

It feels so wrong that we're having to resort to this.

'I've found this consultant in London.' She points to her screen. 'We could just book a one-off appointment and see if he has any ideas. What do you think?'

I visualise the dingy, windowless boxes where most of my consultants spend their days. By comparison, Dr Kaur's private endocrinology clinic is five-star luxury. On arrival, a concierge – yes, a concierge – in an expensive black suit takes us up to the fifth floor, where we're greeted by a receptionist. I feel like I'm checking into a swanky hotel.

Dr Kaur sits behind a large, old-school oak desk. Soft, pastel-toned canvases of waterlilies hang on the walls and Mum and I are guided to two very comfortable taupe armchairs with fancy studs lining their backs. Most impressive are the large glass windows that hover above the River Thames and offer a panoramic view of the London skyline. Tourists would pay good money for this view. Actually, we're paying good money for it too. An introductory 30-minute consultation with Dr Kaur has set us back £300 and that's just for the privilege of meeting him (no tests included).

From the outset, he's truly charming.

'I want to help you, Tilly,' he says, giving me a sympathetic smile. 'This does fit with a number of endocrine disorders. We can easily arrange a panel of tests.'

I'm somewhat touched, until it hits me that a lot of people would probably want to help me if I gave them £300. Whatever the reason, it's a relief that he's going to look into my case.

'We'll do some bloods today, for conditions such as hypothyroidism, Graves' disease, Addison's disease and diabetes. Then we'll book another appointment for a couple of weeks, to go through the results.'

I want to hug him. Bloods TODAY. A follow-up in TWO WEEKS. This is unheard of.

There's no time for hugs. The phone on Dr Kaur's desk rings. He mutters a 'Yes' to the caller, puts the phone down and then swiftly draws our 30-minute appointment to a close. I make that £10 a minute, with a phone call alerting him that our time slot is over so that not a single free minute is added.

Before we leave his office, Dr Kaur pulls something out of his drawer and stretches over his desk.

'If you wouldn't mind just popping your card in.'

Am I seeing things? Is that a card machine? While we're all aware this is a private practice, I kind of assumed the payment would be dealt with more tastefully by Dr Kaur's secretary after the appointment.

'Did he think we were going to do a runner in the few steps between his office and reception?' I whisper to Mum as we leave.

'You can't put a price on your health,' people say, but it turns out that actually you can.

While I await my endocrinology results, an offer of an in-person counselling appointment, with an actual human being, lands in my inbox. I'm not sure what I've done to warrant such a sought-after meeting, but I decide I have to seize the opportunity.

The 'mental-health space' I arrive at today is an ugly, prefab building attached to the main hospital, plonked in the middle of a grey, concrete car park. It looks like it was only ever meant to be a temporary measure but is somehow still standing ten years on.

Inside, the waiting room is crammed full of people sitting on plastic chairs covered in stains and cracks. Most of these people are scrolling through their phones. One man is bashing his hand against the ancient vending machine, frustrated that his KitKat

Chunky is stuck. The air is stale. The atmosphere is claustrophobic. I head to the reception desk.

'Name,' the woman utters, without looking up.

'Tilly Rose,' I smile.

'Take a seat.' She flicks her hand in the direction of the chairs while continuing to stare ahead at her screen. All the chairs are taken. I opt to lean against the far wall, my weak body struggling to stand. I examine the torn posters Blu-Tacked onto the peeling paintwork opposite. One informs me that approximately '45.8 million people in the UK report experiencing common mental-health problems'. Beside this is a pine door, its rectangular slit of glass providing a glimpse into an empty office. Someone has stuck an A4 sheet of paper onto it, with a message scrawled in red permanent marker: 'CLOSED due to staff sickness'.

I think of Dr Kaur's lavish state-of-the-art clinic, with its natural light, lush plants and soft furnishings. This space is by contrast suffocating. The staff working here day in, day out are no doubt part of the 45.8 million.

I nervously peel a strip of skin off my cuticle. Opening up doesn't come easily to me. My head feels dizzy and foggy. I'm boiling hot, my flank stabs and that now-familiar nausea envelops me. I can't really see how talking alone is going to fix any of this but it's got to beat a PowerPoint presentation. At least a counsellor can actually reply to me. I'm prepared to keep an open mind.

After around 40 minutes, a lady called Jane calls my name. She greets me with a friendly smile and I silently wonder whether this environment will eventually take that smile from her. She invites me into a tiny boxroom and asks me to sit down. I kind of expect her to be in one of those curved, cream-leather tilt chairs they always show in therapy scenes in films. Instead, she awkwardly perches on the edge of a dark-blue office swivel chair that has a big tear in it with foam poking through. It's jammed at an awkward height, meaning she's looming down over me.

'First of all, this is a safe space. Everything you say here today is entirely confidential.'

I look over at the flappy white slat blinds lining the glass screen out to the corridor. I count four of the slats have fallen down. What I *say* might be confidential, but the fact that I'm *here*, well, it seems that's fair game.

Jane has a kind, open demeanour and soft voice.

'Could you maybe tell me, in your own words, why you feel you're here today?'

I immediately jump into my years of undiagnosed active tuberculosis, 18 months of treatment and finally getting my life back.

'It was all going so well; my life had transformed. But recently loads of weird symptoms have started to appear again.'

'And emotionally how do you feel about that?'

'Not great,' I say, still smiling.

'I notice you're smiling a lot while telling me about some very difficult times.'

I've got so used to sharing my story as if it's happening to someone else.

'The first time I ended up in hospital, sure, I could fall apart and crumble; but when hospital becomes a way of life, well, I'd have permanently been in a state of crumble.' I give a slight laugh.

Jane asks me to describe the symptoms I'm currently experiencing. She writes them down.

'What about anxiety? Do you ever feel stressed or anxious?'

I'm scared that if I admit to being down or snappy or irritable, Jane will label me with 'anxiety' and it will make it way too easy for the doctors to put everything down to stress. They won't look for anything else.

'I do but these feelings definitely came alongside my other, *physical* symptoms.'

'And what does this stress feel like?'

'I've thought about this quite a bit. It's like someone's repeatedly crocheting my insides and, every so often, they tug at the thread and an intense feeling of anxiety overwhelms me for no reason.'

'That's a very vivid, helpful description. Thank you, Tilly. May I ask, is this in any way affecting your relationships?'

'Yes, it's all stopping me from being *me*. I'm too drained to hang out with my friends or partner. I just want to be in bed the whole time. That's not me.' I know she's wanting me to focus on the emotional stuff but I can't stop myself from adding, 'I feel so ill.'

'Right and do you feel this anxiety is getting better or worse?'

'I feel like *everything* is getting worse. In the last few weeks, I crashed my car because I had a funny turn. I tried doing the mental-health PowerPoint exercises but I couldn't focus. I ended up opening up to my partner about what's going on. Recently, I've been staying with my parents, as I've been too ill to manage on my own when my partner's at work. My mum arranged for me to see an endocrinologist last week. He's run some tests.' This all comes out in a quick gabble.

'And how has this made you feel?'

'Well, I'm kind of hoping the doctor finds something to explain how ill I'm feeling.'

My head is pressured and sore. This is actually harder work than a PowerPoint. You don't have to reply to a screen.

'Right, I think I've begun to work out what's going on here,' Jane says, as our session draws to a close. Relief floods through me. Jane thinks she's cracked my case. This is the moment I've been waiting for.

'I think you are so used to living with illness that you've become trapped in this mindset.'

I tilt my head to the side, unsure what she's getting at.

'It's time to adapt to life as a *well* person, Tilly.'

PATIENT SURVIVAL TIPS

- There's only so much one person can take. Don't beat yourself up if something small tips you over the edge.
- Your partner is choosing to be with *you*. Don't make decisions for them.
- Many private doctors also work in the public sector. You're paying for speed and a swanky waiting room but it's often the same brain.
- If someone suggests your symptoms are down to 'stress' (and you don't agree), pose a few logical questions: 'So, just to clarify, can stress cause recurrent pneumonia?' 'Can I just check, are you suggesting stress is responsible for my bowel resection?' (That would be some stress . . .)
- People can't help if you never let them in.

13

999

'I think my daughter is going into adrenal crisis,' Mum says down the phone to the GP.

After retreating back to Mum and Dad's, I never made it back to my flat with Finn. My symptoms were escalating so much, I could no longer manage basic day-to-day tasks. With Finn being out at work, we made the decision it was best for me to stay at my parents'. All that independence I was relishing has now been snatched away. For the last month, I've led my life from bed. I hated having to email Lewis to tell him I needed time off but when I realised I couldn't even muster the energy to send my copy-and-paste messages anymore, I was left with no choice. I implied I'd just caught a 'little bug'. He didn't need to know the truth: that it feels like my whole body is shutting down.

Mum has been trying to tempt me with nutritious homemade dishes, delivered to my room on trays, with thoughtful touches like flowers in little glass jars to brighten my days. At night, she's rubbed essential oils into my stabbing flank. Dad brings me ice packs to cool my burning head and keeps tabs on how much I'm drinking, repeating the importance of staying hydrated. I've reverted to being a child again, with every need catered for. I'm loved and nurtured and cared for but still, I can't escape my symptoms. Jane's advice is futile. How can I 'adapt to life as a well person' when I don't *feel* well?

Last night, things really escalated. I woke at 3am with excruciating pains in my back. By 8am I'd thrown up six times – none of that dry heaving; we're talking the whole bathroom floor covered in vomit. On my 8:30am trip to the toilet, I never made it to my destination. Instead, Mum found me lying in a heap on the hall floor, crying out with pain in my lower back and legs, repeatedly retching, my body drenched in sweat and simultaneously erupting into goosebumps.

'Tilly saw an endocrinologist two weeks ago and is currently awaiting the results. One of the tests he was doing is for Addison's disease. I've looked into it and she now appears to be displaying all the symptoms of adrenal crisis.' I can hear Mum from the hallway on the phone to Dr Murphy.

She comes over and crouches on the floor beside me.

'Tilly . . .' She leans over to stroke my head. I flinch. Her light touch makes me recoil, a sign that I'm really ill. I just need to lie in my ball and concentrate on the pain. Survival mode leaves no room for affection. 'Dr Murphy has said I need to call an ambulance. They'll be able to help you, Tilly.'

Help. Yes, help. I need help.

A lovely nurse called Sukhi once told me that when people are stuck in the wilderness and a rescue helicopter flies over, the sound of someone *attempting* to help them lifts their vital signs and makes them more likely to survive.

I hear Mum on the phone again.

'My GP has told me to call an ambulance for my daughter. They believe she may be going into an adrenal crisis.'

Mum is my rescue helicopter.

'Yes . . . she's breathing.'

I feel my cold breath on my arm. *Alive.*

'Well, yes. She's conscious but she's quite out of it. Not making much sense, a bit confused.' Another pause. 'An hour!'

I bury my head further into the hall floor, pressing my forehead against the carpet.

'Yes, she is breathing but she can't wait an hour. If this is an adrenal crisis, it's a life-threatening medical emergency.'

My body is starting to tremor with light vibrations. It has registered that the rescue helicopter is far, far away.

'Yes she's breathing but . . . Adrenal crisis . . . Coma . . . Death.' Mum's words make me wail out.

It doesn't feel like I'll survive another hour in the wilderness.

She kneels beside me.

'It's OK, Tilly, it's OK. The ambulance is on its way. They'll make you feel better really soon.' Her voice sounds shaky. I'm not sure I believe her. I want to ask when they'll arrive but no words come out, just mouthfuls of acidic saliva.

A few seconds later, I hear a crunch on the gravel outside and the sound of footsteps on the driveway. My tense muscles relax for a moment. The sound of help.

'Hello . . .' A voice I recognise. My heart sinks like an anchor weighing down my body, fixing me to the hall floor. It's George the postman, not the paramedic. 'Oh no, today looks like a day where I'll sign for you,' he calls.

Mum races out.

'Oh, sorry, George, yes please. Bit of an emergency here again.'

Years ago, during one of my pneumonia admissions, George arrived to deliver our post at the same time as an ambulance pulled up in our driveway. Since that day, if we ever have post that needs signing for and we aren't in, George has signed for us, knowing it might just save us one little job. When your life is a cycle of hospital admissions, wards and waiting rooms, a simple trip to the post office becomes a stress and George thought to take that stress away.

By the time the gravel crunches again, my world is spinning. It's hot and cold and shaking and hurting. It's really hurting. Sometimes I'm in the hall, sometimes I'm elsewhere.

'At last,' I hear Mum say.

The scene is blurry. *Siren. Green. Man. Woman. Help.*

They clip something onto my finger and wrap a cuff around my arm.

'Blood pressure . . . very low.' *Green Man.*

My body begins to tremor, my brain is foggy, confused. I'm with them, then I'm not.

'Tilly, we hear you may be suffering from an adrenal crisis. We're going to give you an injection into the muscle to get the steroid into you quickly.' *Green Woman.*

A swift dart into the base of my back. I cry out as a sharp pain sears at the target. It travels down my right leg, like rain collecting in a muddy puddle, before overflowing through wavy inlets down the hill. I breathe in and out, in and out.

By the time we reach the hospital, the scene is fuzzy, like I'm watching a pixilated film. Every so often I glimpse a shadow, a beam of yellow light, the outline of a person, a voice.

'Your daughter is very seriously ill.' A man's words break through my bleary screen.

I drift in and out of the world, somewhere in the twilight zone between life and death.

Two days later, I re-enter the world. My eyes flicker open, taking in the dark room.

'There she is.' Finn grins at the end of my bed. 'Welcome back.'

I turn my head. Mum leans forward, smiling from the blue plastic chair beside me. Dad stands at the end of the bed. The blinds are drawn closed. I can make out a small wooden side table and a door leading to a bathroom. A blood-pressure machine is attached to my arm. A pulse monitor hangs from my index finger. *Hospital*.

'What happened?' I whisper.

'They think you might have something called Addison's disease. Remember, it was on Dr Kaur's list,' Mum says.

Addison's disease . . . Yes, Mum and I spoke about this. We'd agreed I had lots of the symptoms. She'd said it was something to do with the body not producing the steroid hormone that all the organs need to function.

Mum now recounts the last few days to me, how I collapsed on the hall floor, how we arrived here in an ambulance, how the on-call doctor in A&E happened to be an endocrinologist. My little bit of luck.

'He was lovely, Tilly. He pointed over to you and said to me, "This is what an adrenal crisis looks like . . ."'

Adrenal crisis. Coma. Death. It starts to come back.

'Am I going to die?'

'No, you're not going to die. They're treating you with the steroid now. You're going to keep feeling better.' Mum holds my hand.

I tilt my head to the side, trying to work it out. It's too overwhelming. I flop my head back into the pillow, floating in and out of the room and the conversation. At 3pm, my body breaks out into a film of sweat and the pain in my back stabs. My head feels dizzy and sore. I clutch it, returning to my position face down on the bed.

'This keeps happening. An hour before the next steroid IV is due, she gets worse,' I hear Mum say. 'I'm going to ring the call-bell.'

She leans over and presses my buzzer. We wait and wait and wait.

'Hello.' A voice from the doorway. A nurse.

Mum asks her if we can see an endocrinologist.

'It's the weekend,' the nurse says.

'But she keeps going downhill before her next meds are due,' Finn says.

'There's no endocrinologist in the hospital this weekend,' the nurse informs us.

'Well, she needs to see someone. Look at her . . .' Finn gestures over to me, face down, bottom in the air, grimacing in pain.

Three hours later, there's another knock at my door.

'Hello, hello. Right, I've only got a few minutes.' She sounds breathless, rushed. 'I'm Dr Edwards. I'm on A&E today. I've just run up from downstairs but it's full, so I need to get back. There are lots of *really* ill patients.'

This is a line I've heard before. I've now entered a competitive game of 'Guess Who?', hospital style. The doctors assess all the patients and must then decide who's 'the *most* ill' and who's 'the *most* likely to die'. I swallow back my tears, as I realise 'adrenal crisis, coma, death' isn't going to win. Now that I've passed through the doors of A&E, my face card has been flipped down. I'm no longer 'ill enough' to warrant being cared for by a doctor in a hospital. There aren't enough of them to go around.

'Best keep things as they are, until you're reviewed by the endocrinology team on Monday,' Dr Edwards says.

'But we don't even know for certain what's wrong with Tilly yet. We were told they'd be doing a test to check for Addison's disease,' Mum says.

'Yes but we can't do that now,' Dr Edwards says.

'Why not?' Dad asks.

'It's the weekend. We don't do those tests at the weekend.' With that, she races off.

For the next two days, Mum, Dad and Finn help me navigate the wilderness of the weekend ward. Each time the steroid runs out, I begin to deteriorate. On Sunday, a junior doctor swings by. He's like a politician on *Newsnight*, terrified of being quoted, and somehow avoids answering a single one of our questions.

'Is there a consultant we could see?' Dad asks when it becomes clear we're getting nowhere.

'It's the weekend,' Dr No-Comment reminds us.

By the evening, my bin is overflowing. Finn lifts the bag out and hovers in the doorway.

'Is there somewhere I could get rid of this please?' he asks, as a nurse walks past.

'Short on cleaners today. It's the weekend,' she responds.

Finn returns with his arms full of rubbish.

'What were you thinking, Tilly? You really should have timed your adrenal crisis Monday to Friday, preferably between nine and five,' Dad grins.

Even in the worst times, Dad always manages to make me laugh.

After all these years of patient life, I can say with some authority that Tuesdays are hospital goals. Nothing much happens on a Monday. The doctors are all playing catchup. Wednesdays and Thursdays don't leave much time for tests. Tuesdays are when stuff gets done.

Tuesday gets off to a good start. My nurse, Perlah, wakes me at 8am on the dot, ready for my first blood. She's in and out all day, taking timed samples for my Synacthen test (the test for Addison's disease) and rushing them down to the lab.

'How was your weekend?' I ask her, looking away as she inserts the needle into my right arm.

'It was good,' she says. 'I spoke to my children on video call.'

I hold my thumb in my fist as she wriggles the needle.

'Sorry, I have terrible veins,' I say. 'Where are your children?'

'Back in the Philippines. My home.'

I turn to look out of the window. I already miss my own home, only a few miles down the road. Hospital can never feel like home.

'We're in!' she exclaims, gesturing down to my arm.

'Result!' I smile. 'Have they gone back to the Philippines for a holiday?' I ask.

Perlah shakes her head and looks down.

'They live there, with my mum.' Her eyes now fill. 'I haven't seen them for 15 years.'

I take a sharp inhale. *15 years*. My eyes now mirror hers.

'Perlah, that's terrible.'

Grief is painted into the creases in her face, grief for her own children, thousands of miles away; grief for a life that could have been.

'I send them money home. They have a good education because of me.'

'Tell us about them, Perlah,' Mum says.

For the rest of the day, as she takes my blood, Perlah adds more and more snippets, building a picture of her son and daughter. She's so proud that her son is applying to university and her daughter is top of her class at high school. The focus of the conversation remains solely around their education.

'Education is freedom,' she says.

The medics have had to remove my steroid drip for the test and by lunchtime my symptoms are deteriorating. I take this as a sign that Addison's disease seems quite likely. My body seems to love the steroid. I spend the rest of the day lying in my tight ball and let Perlah's words distract me from the pain. As she speaks, an almost dreamy longing radiates from her face. For a short while, as she describes them, a little part of her son and daughter are back with her, in the room.

'I want them to have a better life than me,' she tells us.

'They're lucky to have you, Perlah,' Mum responds.

I look over at my own mum, who never leaves my side, who sleeps in the chair beside me for nights on end, who would do anything for me. What if that 'anything' was moving halfway across the world to give me a better life? I know she'd do it, but I also know it would break her heart.

'From one mother to another . . .' Mum leans over and squeezes Perlah's hand. 'You must miss them so much.'

She nods, wiping a tear from her cheek.

'But I am happy, if they are happy.'

'Do you have any family over here?' Mum asks.

Perlah shakes her head. We learn that she lives in a small flat alone. Her life is a repetitive cycle of working, eating and talking to her children on video call. She spends as little money as possible, sending as much as she can back home. Perlah has given up her own life so that her children can live theirs. She has a few Filipino friends over here who do the same. A culture of selfless love.

'They don't really know me. I'm not a mother to them.'

' "Mother" is a title you earn. You are a mother in the truest sense. You live only for your children,' Mum says.

'One day I will see them again.' I follow her gaze out of the window, onto the concrete car park below.

I know that feeling of living for the future. Perlah is living for when she sees her children again. I am living for when I get better. Sometimes it is only the hope of tomorrow that gets us through today.

PATIENT SURVIVAL TIPS

- Always know what you're currently being tested for.
- The 999-call set emergency questions don't always encompass 'zebras'. If you're diagnosed with a rare condition, register with your local ambulance service so there's a note on file when you call.
- If you could have your heart attack, haemorrhage or broken leg from Monday to Friday, that would be ideal.
- Sometimes laughter is the best medicine of all.
- Everyone has a story. Sometimes you just need to ask.

14

STRIPES

I am becoming a zebra with way too many stripes. On Wednesday morning, the consultant endocrinologist confirms that Mum is right: the Synacthen test has proved that I have Addison's disease.

'Addison's disease is where the adrenal glands are impaired, which means the body cannot produce cortisol,' Dr Zhao tells me. 'Cortisol is needed for every organ to function.'

If only Dr Kaur's tests had come through earlier, this crisis could have been avoided.

'You will have to take replacement steroid medication at set times, four times a day, for the rest of your life.'

Forever. My life is about to change *forever.*

'If you don't take it, you could go into a crisis like you had last week. This can lead to a dramatic drop in blood pressure, a coma and death.'

It would be nice to slowly get used to the idea that I now have a rare and lifelong disease before focusing on the absolute worst-case scenario.

'Let's look on the bright side,' I say, swallowing back my tears.

Mum squishes up next to me on the bed, holding me in her arms.

'I'm sorry, Tilly. It's a lot to take in – but now we know what it is, we can focus on getting you better, can't we, Dr Zhao?' I can feel Mum willing her to say something comforting. She says nothing, just gives a brief nod.

'This will also explain your skin pigmentation.' She points to my upper lip. The tanned moustache Mum keeps trying to convince me 'you can barely see' is clearly very visible. 'It leads to an increase in melanin and means patients often look very healthy when they are actually very ill.'

Maybe the one plus will be having a golden glow for the rest of my life.

'It's also quite common for patients to have "mini-crises" that go undiagnosed before they have their first proper one,' Dr Zhao continues, as if she's giving a presentation to a roomful of doctors, not a frightened mother and daughter who had a close shave with death last week. 'Have you had any?'

'Earlier this year, I had a similar episode. A&E dismissed me as just being drunk but I'd barely drunk anything. It never made any sense. Do you think that was one?' I whisper.

'Yes, it's likely. Patients are often misdiagnosed as being drunk. Crises can make you confused, unable to walk and experience difficulty communicating.'

I feel sick thinking back to that night. How differently it could have ended.

Mum hugs me harder.

'You're lucky really. We diagnose some Addison's patients at the autopsy,' Dr Zhao says.

Autopsy. My eyes widen in panic. Mum wraps her arm around my head, forming a protective guard between Dr Zhao's words and me.

'They've found it now, Tilly,' she says. 'So that's not you.'

You've found it, I think, squeezing Mum's hand. I lean further into her chest, feeling her heartbeat against my skin. A heart that beats for me day and night, however old I get. Dr Zhao's right. I am lucky. I am lucky to have Mum.

'Why do I have Addison's disease?' I ask.

'We're not 100 per cent sure from the tests so far.'

Story of my life.

'But TB can be a cause of Addison's disease, so that's our working assumption.'

I think back to the farm, the cow, the milk – something so inconspicuous, which has altered my entire path.

'Anyway, if you take your daily steroids you should be able to live a relatively normal life,' Dr Zhao says casually, like she's advising I just pop a few paracetamol.

After she leaves, I ask Mum to give me a moment alone. I need some space to wrap my head around all of this before calling Finn to share the news. Mum pops outside to call Dad and Auntie. I lie on the bed, swaying from side to side, clutching a pillow to my tummy. Hugging it brings a sort of comfort. A numbness travels from my brain, down through my limbs. The tears can come later. For now, I need to take the time to understand how it all fits together: I have Addison's disease. My body does not produce cortisol. Cortisol is needed to live. I will have to take steroid tablets at timed intervals every day for the rest of my life. If I miss my meds, I could go into an 'adrenal crisis'. The doctors will give me IV steroids to treat this. If it's left too late, I could go into a coma. I could die.

'*Some patients are diagnosed at the autopsy . . .*' Dr Zhao's words echo through me, vibrating through my limbs. They shake my very foundations, reducing me to a wet mess of loud, uncontrollable tears, breathless, hiccuping sobs and intermittent wails.

Mum hears me from the corridor and races in. She holds me in her arms, kissing the top of my head.

'Half the battle is knowing what it is, Tilly. We knew you were ill. Now we can do everything within our power to make you better.'

When my tears finally settle, I contemplate Mum's words. Without a diagnosis, I've been trapped in the forest, concealed under the overgrown foliage. A diagnosis means someone has, finally, untangled the branches. I can now step out of the shadows. I am no longer hidden from view in the odyssey of the 'undiagnosed'. Mum has pulled me from the wilderness. I now have a label and there is a clear path out.

On day ten of this admission, the steroid seems to have finally penetrated my system enough to give me the energy to shower. I kind of want to send Sue, the mental-health assessor, a pic of my big moment.

'We're going to have to sort this hair,' Mum says.

My go-to hospital hairstyle is usually a neat plait but this time I arrived in an emergency and was far too ill to give my hair a second thought. Ten days of lying on it has now resulted in a matted bird's nest at the back of my head, locked in impenetrable knots. Mum tries brushing, combing, wetting, conditioning and even smothering it in oil. Nothing works. In the end, she resorts to the scissors.

'There are chunks that are so stuck together I'm going to have to cut them, Tilly.'

Over the last week, the medics have pumped me so full of steroids and fluids that my face is bulging, my wrists are so swollen my bracelets are bursting off, my rings are stuck on my fingers, and let's not forget my blotchy moustache. I'm already panicking that my appearance has taken a real turn and now we're throwing a serious bad-hair day (month) into the mix.

'You're beautiful to me,' Finn keeps saying each night when he visits after work.

I look at the chunks of hair now falling to the floor as Mum hacks away.

'The fluid will go as soon as they stop the drips and your hair will grow back. These are things that aren't worth worrying about.'

I attempt to organise my mind into a) stuff that *really is* worth stressing about (for example, having an illness that threatens to kill me without warning); and b) stuff that is irrelevant (for example, having a bad-hair day). I try to shelve the minor stuff, telling myself these things don't matter. And yet, much to my annoyance, the 'bad-hair day' stress somehow finds a way to keep coming back, smothering the 'life-threatening illness' stress. Deep down, I know that going on and on about my hair is a way of expressing a graver fear that's harder to talk about. 'I hate my hair,' is easier to say than, 'I'm scared this illness will kill me.' So, for today, I choose to keep the irrelevant stress alive, torturing myself by repeatedly heading to the mirror.

Day 11 is discharge day. I'm so excited at the prospect of making my great escape but there's one thing that still doesn't feel right.

'My head pain is still excruciating,' I say to the junior doctor, Caro, this morning. I've asked every day if someone could look into it before I leave. 'Could it possibly be scanned?'

'There are *really* ill patients who need scans.' Caro has clearly done her training under Dr Edwards and Dr Zhao and has honed her 'Guess Who?' tactics. Discharge day means my face card doesn't get a look in and has instantly been flipped down. I'm at the bottom of their priority list, nowhere near 'ill enough' to warrant a scan anymore.

'It's just we've read that if pain puts your body under physical stress, it can trigger an adrenal crisis,' I say. With the constant talk of death, comas and autopsies, I question how ill you have to be, in order to be worthy of a scan.

'You'd need to be seen by a neurologist first,' Caro says.

'OK great, so can I be?' I've been clutching my searing right eyebrow for over a week and constantly placing ice packs on my pressured head. It feels like it's about to explode. Taking the steroid initially calmed it a little but it's now continuing to dominate every second of the day. It distracts from anything I try to do. Holding a conversation, reading a book or watching TV have all become impossible. I can do nothing but think about the pain.

'There isn't a neurologist in the hospital.'

'No neurologist in the whole hospital?'

Caro shakes her head. Where does that leave all the patients having strokes and seizures? The autopsy, I guess.

'The pharmacy will be up soon to arrange your discharge meds,' she says, swiftly changing the subject. With that, she rushes out of the room.

I push my fingers deep into my right eyebrow, rubbing and needling and pressing the agonising spot. Sometimes pain distracts from pain.

A few hours later, a pharmacist called Devi arrives at the end of my bed.

'First up,' she says, 'have you managed to source a medical-alert bracelet?'

'I haven't been told I needed one.'

'You need to wear one at all times. It has to have this universal medical-alert symbol on.' She points to a picture on her phone of a six-pointed star. In its centre, a snake is wrapped around a thin rod. 'This is called the Rod of Asclepius. He's the god of medicine and healing.'

Asclepius sounds like a pretty great guy to have wrapped around my wrist.

'You also need to get the bracelet engraved with the name of your condition,' Devi adds. 'That way, if you're ever in an accident or unable to communicate, the paramedics or anyone who comes across you will know that you have a medical condition requiring specific treatment.'

It was believed that Asclepius had the ability to resurrect and heal those teetering on the edge of death, but that power now seems quite dependent on someone actually recognising his magical rod. I think of all my years of being a patient and how, until this conversation, I had no idea this was the universal 'medical alert' symbol. Somehow, I need to get Asclepius on the map.

Devi now hands me a white paper bag.

'We've put some extra packets of steroid in, just in case you need to follow the sick-day rule before your next appointment.'

I stare up at her blankly.

'What's the sick-day rule?'

'It's part of your emergency procedure.'

'What emergency procedure?' I ask.

'Has nobody explained this to you?'

I shake my head. Devi's face displays a mixture of surprise and concern. She perches down on the chair next to me.

'It's really important you understand this, Tilly,' she says, before going on to carefully explain that when a 'normal' person, with functioning adrenal glands, is unwell or under stress, their own body *automatically* produces more cortisol. Patients with Addison's disease don't produce *any* cortisol, so if we are unwell or under stress we have to *double* our steroid medication to compensate. Just a bit of lifesaving info that no one thought worth mentioning.

'If you don't, you can risk descending into an adrenal crisis and we don't want that again, do we?' Devi says.

The distressing image of me sprawled on the hall floor bursts into my mind.

'Now, the lifesaving emergency injection,' she says. 'All Addison's patients *must* carry this with them 24/7. If you start to display symptoms of an adrenal crisis you must be injected with a vial of hydrocortisone *immediately*.'

She advises us to practise administering it on an orange – a fun 'around the fruit bowl' activity for my return home.

'If you are ever vomiting and can't keep down your tablets, you *must* use the injection and then call an ambulance straightaway.'

I inwardly shudder.

'This injection could save your life so I can't stress enough: you must *always* have it with you.'

Mum's writing down everything Devi says in her notepad, so we have all the instructions back home.

'Thank you, Devi, that's really helpful to know. Can I see the injection?' I ask.

She pauses for a moment and looks a bit awkward.

'I'm afraid . . . we don't actually have one.'

I see the confusion spread across Mum's face.

'Sorry, Devi, are you saying you don't have the lifesaving injection for Tilly to take home?'

'Unfortunately, we don't have one in the hospital.'

'You don't have one?' I repeat back.

Devi looks down awkwardly. I sense she has been put in an impossible position.

'No, we don't.'

'So, what do I do?'

'I suggest you book an appointment with your GP as soon as possible and arrange to get one from them.'

I lock eyes with Mum, in absolute disbelief.

PATIENT SURVIVAL TIPS

- If it gives you the chance to have a good moan, then sometimes it can be helpful to pin scarier emotions onto trivial stresses.
- A neat plait is your bedridden hair's best friend.
- New diagnoses can be overwhelming; be sure to ask all your questions before you're discharged.
- Rare diseases are not always widely understood. It's time for you to become the 'expert patient'.
- Be aware of the medical-alert symbol: ✳ Knowing this could save a life!

15

TRAUMA

Storms are usually fleeting. They rumble for a while, then build up to a dramatic crescendo and explode. In the aftermath, it takes time and effort to clear the path; but one day, the sun peeps through the clouds and patches of blue appear again. I thought that first adrenal crisis was the biggest storm I'd have to weather. Instead, I'm stuck in perpetual sleet and snowstorm with no promise of blue skies ahead.

In the two years since being diagnosed with Addison's disease, the emergency injection – the one I was discharged home *without*, that we had to source *ourselves* – has been used over 20 times. Dr Zhao's forecast of a 'relatively normal life' didn't include these persistent weather warnings. The steroids don't seem to touch my body. I pop them like sweets and, in a desperate bid to control my escalating symptoms, the doses are becoming increasingly higher. The doctors keep telling me I should be clinically obese (high steroids usually = weight gain) but instead, I'm withering away. The storm lives on, striking down more and more areas of my life in its wake.

Today, I make the decision to give up my recruitment job. Actually, that's not right. I have been *forced* to give up my recruitment job. Chronic illness leaves no choice. I'm certainly not made for recruitment – in fact I'm terrible at it – so after putting down the phone to Lewis, I'm surprised by the feeling of intense sadness that envelops me. I lie on my bed, staring up at my gold Ikea lampshade, and mull it all over. I realise I'm not mourning the role itself but rather the 'normal' life it represents. Resigning makes me face a stark reality: I'm once again too ill to maintain a 'proper job'.

'At least I still have my student platform,' I say to Finn.

The truth is, I'm fed up living a life of 'at leasts':

'I had to give up recruitment but at least I have my own project . . .'

'I missed Phoebe's birthday but at least I made it to Liv's drinks . . .'

'I ended up in hospital for two days but at least it wasn't a week . . .'

Bargaining with myself has become a way to get through. Any small win becomes a reason to celebrate, but I can't help grieving all the things I've lost to this illness. It's like a thief that's returned to my life and is intent on robbing me of one thing I'll never get back: moments in time. I dream of being spontaneous, responding to every invite with a big 'Yes' and choosing what I do with my days. Instead, this cruel illness dictates that everything has to be carefully balanced and planned. Take a weekend away: my friends can grab a rucksack and go. I, instead, spend hours arranging prescriptions, packing meds, printing emergency protocols, navigating travel plans and stressing over whether I'll even manage to power through once I arrive. To hold onto a semblance of normality, I push myself to turn up at certain events, so desperate to feel part of something beyond all of this, but it's a struggle. Chronic illness changes the threshold; I'll find myself in a room at a party, knowing that if a healthy person felt this ill, they wouldn't even consider getting out of bed. I might be there, smiling, but so many happy times have started to feel like moments to endure, memories forever tainted.

A lot of the time, I simply have to turn these invites down. 'Tilly's unwell again,' people say when I miss another party, another holiday, another event. They don't always stop to think what it means; how much worse it is when it keeps happening.

This week, the gusty winds whistle and howl and eventually become so turbulent they land me right back in A&E, in *another* adrenal attack. It's time for my usual 48 hours of IV steroid, guaranteed to turn the menacing storm into a gentle breeze.

Finn is sitting beside me on the familiar hard, turquoise chair.

'The girls have all been messaging to see how you are.'

Once I finally received my Addison's diagnosis, I found it easier to share with my friends. A new label at least provided me with an explanation. It made a lot of sense to everyone I told, given TB is one of the causes of Addison's disease. What doesn't make sense is why I *keep* going into crisis.

'It just doesn't happen,' the doctors tell me again and again.

Trust me, it does.

I stare down at the yellow and purple bruises creating a tapestry of old and new across my skin. The scars from the past admission haven't yet faded and already fresh threads of pain have been added to the patchwork.

Finn flicks up his phone and begins reading out some of the messages from my friends. First there's one from Phoebe:

So unbelievably shit that you are back in Tills ☹

This is what I want to hear. Recently, when the girls said they felt helpless and didn't know what to do, I decided it was time to tell them. They can't change the situation but they can acknowledge how rubbish it is and how much the FOMO hurts. Rather than skirting around the subject or going silent and awkward, they now address it head on. We're all closer for it.

'Then a classic from Liv,' Finn laughs, reading her message. 'She wants to know, "Can you have alcohol in hospital?"' He puts his fingers in quote marks.

Like I know it's not encouraged but if you say just had a broken leg and it was Friday night, could someone bring you in a prosecco?

I crack up. Liv always knows how to make me laugh. For a few blissful minutes this is the perfect distraction. Finn takes a photo of the bag of fluids hanging from my drip stand. We ping it over to her.

Sodium chloride will have to do for Friday night #HospitalStyle

I look over at Finn now, armed with a bag containing magazines, juices, tissues, earplugs, hand san, face wipes, dry shampoo and a room spray. I may have become the expert patient but those around me have also become expert carers. They know what I need, without me even asking.

I lean over and hold Finn's hand. He kisses me lightly on the forehead. It should be a beautiful, tender moment, but on the other side of the curtain Bed 6 has raging diarrhoea and is reliant on a commode.

'I'll be back in five minutes,' I hear the healthcare assistant say.

Ten minutes later, the healthcare assistant still hasn't returned.

'Please, please,' the lady in Bed 6 calls out.

She sounds distressed. I assure her through the curtain that I've pressed my call-bell on her behalf. When nobody emerges, Finn heads off in search of help. Thirty minutes later, my poor neighbour is still waiting. She's now crying, having spent over half an hour sitting in a bowl of her own diarrhoea, abandoned in the middle of a communal ward. She's faced the indignity of this playing out live in front of a bay of other patients who can hear and smell it all. I feel so sad for her, knowing what it feels like to be reliant on the various stages of the hierarchical hospital toilet structure:

1. **Your own toilet.** Your diarrhoea is so bad, you are considered an *infection risk*. The day the diarrhoea subsides can be a sad one, resulting in a return to the communal ward.
2. **Communal bathroom.** You can pretty much guarantee one of your ward pals will have left behind a nice gift.

There seems to be an unwritten rule, for some, that as soon as they're admitted to hospital they should no longer have to use a toilet brush – they're *ill*, remember.

3. **Commode.** Dictionary definition: 'a piece of furniture containing a concealed chamber pot'. This is a really nice way to describe the portable potty embedded within a plastic chair that is easily accessible from your bed. The sounds and smells are also easily accessible – to *everyone*.

4. **Bedpan.** Dictionary definition: 'a receptacle used by a bedridden patient for urine and faeces'. Imagine being asked to lie down flat, then being asked to piss.

5. **Nappy.** Dictionary definition: 'a piece of towelling or other absorbent material wrapped round a baby's bottom and between its legs to absorb and retain urine and faeces'. The dictionary is wrong. 'Who needs their nappy changing?' is, sadly, a phrase I have regularly heard bandied around the adult wards, where – I can assure you – there are no babies.

Note: If you are given the luxury of Options 1 or 2, count your blessings.
Extra note: Use the loo brush.

There's always a bit of potluck when it comes to whether I'll be allowed an overnight companion by my side in hospital. For some ward sisters it's an instant no, whereas others hear 'rare disease' and feel safer having a family member around. Thankfully, tonight's ward sister, Mia, falls into the latter category and allows Mum to stay next to me in the Acute Medical Unit (AMU). Lots of things remain uncertain but one thing I can confirm is that she will get absolutely no sleep. It's just as noisy and chaotic as A&E because AMU basically *is* A&E. Think of it like an extension built on the side, to house the overflow. By moving me to AMU precisely three hours and fifty-eight minutes after I arrive, the hospital continue to meet their A&E waiting-time targets. AMU is the ultimate holding bay, a way to cheat the system while the doctors work out what to do or where to put you. I always seem to have 'AMU' written all over me.

I glance over at Mum's silhouette, contorting between the hard wooden arms of the hospital chair, and feel that familiar twist of guilt.

'You are so loved,' she whispers, squeezing my shoulder.

Mum has lived her life in that chair and made my life better by doing so.

Just as we're settling down, a man bobs his head around my curtain and holds up an A4 sheet of paper.

'Before you go to sleep, we need to fill out a property list.'

It's midnight. I pause for a second to take in the torturous screams, bleeping monitors and irritating hum of machines. Midnight or not, sleep isn't on the cards.

'Of course. No problem,' I smile.

He switches on the light above my bed. Mum uncurls herself from the chair and sits upright. While I could not care less if I lose my white T-shirt that only earlier today was splatted with blood as my cannula was inserted, the hospital is clearly terrified that I could later sue if it went missing. Consequently, this man at the end of my bed insists on knowing every single belonging I have with me – and I mean *everything*.

'Do you have a bra?'

'Erm, yes, I'm wearing one . . .'

'Knickers?'

'Wearing those too.'

He ticks a few boxes. I'm now cringing as I realise he didn't need to know their whereabouts, only that I have them. It's midnight on the open ward and I'm openly sharing with anyone listening that no one should fret: I am *wearing* my underwear.

'What about other belongings?'

'The only thing of any real value is my phone,' I say, hoping to bring the conversation to an end.

'Valuables must be locked in this side cabinet for safekeeping.' He gestures to the top drawer.

I nod. This will not be happening. I know the safest place for my phone is in my bed, glued to my side at all times.

'What about this?' He points to my floral notepad.

This property list is proving to be more thorough than any medical examination I've had since arriving here. After I've named every piece of clothing and underwear from top to bottom and we've gone through all the items piled in my messy handbag, the man only takes his leave when I tell him about my most valuable possession of all: my rose quartz stone. The spiritual life clearly isn't for him and he finally asks for my signature, confirming that the loss or damage of any of these items is my sole responsibility. I must obligingly accept that even if I am bedbound, incapacitated or potentially unconscious, if someone steals my rose quartz there will be no hospital search party looking into its disappearance.

A while later, another voice bounces through my curtain.

'Someone needs your bed.'

I glance at my phone. It's now 1:30am. Mum looks across at me. Of course, we're both still wide awake.

'I'm Ken.' The man pokes his head in.

Under any other circumstances in life, if a man called Ken entered my room at 1:30am and plucked me from my bed it would be totally acceptable to scream for help or call the police. But this Ken is a hospital porter and somehow that makes it OK.

'I thought I was staying here?'

Nurse Mia now pokes her head around.

'Someone needs this bed now, so you're on the move.'

I'm pretty certain there are hundreds of beds in this hospital. Why does this patient need this exact bed, the one I am currently sleeping in?

'No chance they could have waited until morning . . .?' I grin.

Ken reminds me that he is simply the messenger. This decision lay in the hands of the *bed managers*.

Every expert patient knows it is the bed managers who ultimately decide your fate. They are a subset of mythical creatures who have an omniscient presence over every ward. They decide just how hellish your sleepover is going to be. Will you be given a side room (aka VIP hospital luxury) or be condemned to communal living? Will you be assigned a roomful of screamers or sleepers? Will you end up on Ward 18 (currently undergoing 'investigation') or Ward 7 (Platinum Award for high standards)?

You hear of them in hushed whispers, across wards, through corridors, on the end of phones: 'The bed manager says she needs her own room . . .' 'The bed manager says we need to find someone to discharge . . .' 'The bed manager says he's not ill enough to stay here anymore . . .'

The wards are always at overcapacity, which means the bed managers are tasked with the never-ending job of searching for beds. At times, their decisions seem to defy logic but there is no chance of finding them to discuss. Contrary to their name, they are never at your bedside.

'You can always take it up with PALS [Patient Advice & Liaison Service, aka complaint hotline],' Ken says.

'Wheel me there right now . . .' I joke.

He looks at me like I've lost it.

'It will have to wait. It's 1:30am. Everyone is asleep.'

Exactly, Ken, exactly.

Meanwhile, Mum springs from her chair and begins gathering up my bags, placing them on my bed. She's now adept at this sort of speedy middle-of-the-night departure.

'Where's Tilly moving to?' Mum asks, as we exit the bay, into the corridor, where Mia is stationed.

'Ward 9,' Mia mutters, while continuing to scroll her phone.

'Do they understand about Tilly's Addison's disease?' asks Mum.

'Yes, yes,' Mia responds.

'Do they know about her emergency procedure?'

'Handover will all be done, Mum, don't you worry.'

I glance down at the desk. Mia is too busy perusing an online shopping website for her summer wardrobe to bother looking up.

Within moments, I am being wheeled out of AMU and into the bright lights of the freezing-cold corridor, before finally being dropped off at the destination the bed managers have deemed most suitable: the gastroenterology ward.

Naturally, I have zero gastro symptoms.

Ken wheels me into a cubicle in the corner of a four-person bay. It's dark and difficult to get my bearings but it seems quiet at least. I'll never get used to being in hospital but, like anything else, the more times I experience it, the less shocking it becomes. It still hurts but I'm learning to grow a thicker skin, in order to cope, in order to survive. Now I'm on a proper ward, Mum is made to leave. Surviving alone is always more daunting.

'Before I go, Tilly, shall we just check they definitely know about your Addison's disease and emergency protocol?'

We ask to speak to the ward sister, Hazel, and talk in hushed whispers around the bed.

'Yes, we know about your condition from the handover,' Hazel nods. 'You have Edison's disease.'

'Addison's disease?' I clarify, assuming I've misheard her.

'Yes, Edison's disease.'

'Sorry, what is Edison's disease?'

She stares at me blankly. It turns out, Hazel doesn't know what 'Edison's disease' is because 'Edison's disease' doesn't exist.

After clearing up this potentially fatal breakdown in communication and giving a 2am show-and-tell presentation of my emergency-injection kit, Mum reluctantly prepares to take her leave. She writes 'ADDISON'S DISEASE' on a piece of paper in red permanent marker and balances it on the table at the end of my bed. She lays my injection kit next to me in the bed and then rubs my rose quartz stone between her fingers and places it in my palm.

'All my good energy is in there for you,' she says, squeezing my hand.

'I'll be fine, Mum. As long as I have my emergency injection, nothing can go wrong.'

She looks over her shoulder all the way down the corridor to the ward exit, until the heavy double doors shut behind her.

My new nurse, Leo, turns off the lamp above my bed.

'Goodnight,' he says, exiting the bay.

I put in my earplugs and roll over, clutching my stone to chest. Just as I start to drift off to sleep, a horrible waft descends over my bed. I wonder if I'm imagining it to start with. The smell gets worse, becoming a stench that engulfs me. It is so strong it is tangible, like smoke suffocating my airways and filling my lungs.

I press my call-bell. Nobody comes.

I lie cocooned in a ball, holding my nose and desperately trying to breathe through my mouth. This isn't a normal hospital smell. Something bad is happening in the next bed and nobody knows. I switch on the light above my bed and cry out as the floor comes into view. Spilling from under Bed 2's curtain and clawing its way towards me is a river of blood. Within touching distance, a silent, volcanic eruption is taking place. The lava is snaking its way out of an actual human body and drowning my bed in its wake. I want to run but I am attached to so many drips and monitors I can't escape. I press my bell again. This time I call out.

Leo pokes his head into the bay.

'Sorry, love, just got caught with—' The stench hits him.

Within seconds, the ward becomes a frenzy of bleeps, alarms, buzzers and footsteps. Hordes of staff gather around Bed 2.

'She's losing litres of blood,' the consultant explains to the team, before firing instructions on the emergency procedure.

It feels as though I am in the centre of a horror film and yet, by some miracle, every member of staff remains steadfastly calm. It is as if the consultant has told them they are standing in litres of cherry aid, not bodily fluids.

I manoeuvre myself to the chair, where I huddle my knees to my chest, silent tears rolling down my cheeks, rocking back and forth in a desperate attempt to block it all out.

I glance over at the team and I am in awe. I realise they've spent their whole careers preparing for this moment. The doctors have gone to medical school, the nurses have gone to uni – but what about the patients?

No one ever sat me down and said, 'Here's the manual on how to cope when, at 3am, the patient in the bed next to you dies of a bowel haemorrhage.'

I am directed to a hard plastic chair in the corridor. The bright lights shine down on me. The blood-stained river soaking the floor is no longer within my sight but it is there haunting my mind. Metres away I can hear the cleanup begin. Instructions fly across the room.

The stench wafts through the air, a physical reminder that death now lingers on the ward. I want to be held. I want Mum here, enveloping me in her arms, stroking my hair, telling me that I will get through this, but I am no longer a child. Adults are expected to cope with this alone. I hug myself, wrapping my arms around my knees, squeezing my own body as tightly as I can. Tears begin to trickle down my cheeks. Within moments, irrepressible sobs burst out. I cry and I cry until my chest aches and my tummy burns.

I once read an article about extreme neglect in a children's home. The investigating journalist entered a room filled with cot upon cot of newborn babies. He was struck by one thing. It was silent. Babies are meant to cry. It is their way of telling the world that they need feeding or changing or that they are in pain. It is an instinctive human communication and yet babies also learn that there is no point in crying if no one responds.

Tonight, I am the baby in the cot. Staff walk up and down the corridor, past my chair. None of them look at me. None of them come near me. I cry myself into silence.

At 4:30am, a nurse calls from the desk.

'Were you Bed 1?'

I nod.

'You can go back now.'

I unfurl from my ball and stand up. My legs feel shaky. I hold onto the wall as I make my way back up the corridor. The strong smell of disinfectant fills my airways. A wave of nausea rises in my chest. I hover at the entrance to the bay. The floor has been scrubbed, the bed has been changed, everything looks as it was. In just a few hours, a new patient will lie in Bed 2, the sun will shine through the window at dawn and a new day will begin. The doctors will enter for the morning ward round. It will be like nothing has changed and yet everything has changed. I have now seen death and it is something I will never be able to unsee.

PATIENT SURVIVAL TIPS

- When people ask what they can do to support you, *tell them!* Most people want to help, they just don't always know how.
- You have different friends for different things. When times are tough, you need the person you can cry to but also the person who makes you laugh. You need the person who listens but also the one who distracts with their own entertaining tales. You need the person you can chill on the sofa with but also the one who takes you out and lets you dream of happier times.
- The hospital 'property list' may well be more thorough than any medical examination. Don't pack for a week's holiday and don't bring anything weird.
- When a porter arrives to move you to a new ward, before you leave, ask where you are being taken and check your treatment plan has been written up.
- It is brave to feel. Adults are also allowed to crumble. Sometimes you need to cry.

16

STOP

The next morning, Mum, Dad and Finn hold me close but I know that no amount of hugging can take away the cold mist of death that now lingers on every surface and in every crevice of the ward. It clings to me like a sticky film, making my skin clammy and my limbs tremble. Addison's disease is all about the body's inability to produce the stress hormone cortisol. Patients are sometimes advised to pop an extra steroid tablet when giving a particularly stressful presentation at work. I wonder what they advise you take in the aftermath of witnessing the person next to you die a cruel and gruesome death. I suppose there's no precedent for that.

As soon as the day shift arrive on duty, I immediately ask to be moved to a different ward, calmly explaining the events of the previous night.

'That's not possible,' I am told again and again.

After pleading and getting absolutely nowhere, I decide there is only so much one body and one mind can take. I cannot endure another second overlooking Bed 2. I decide I'll take high dose steroid tablets to compensate. My poor little adrenal glands are safer off at home. I do something I have never done before and hope never to do again. I self-discharge.

When it comes down to it, all this actually involves is signing a brief form absolving the hospital of any responsibility if I die beyond their doors. I have to assert that this is 100 per cent my own decision. This isn't strictly true, of course. I never decided to be a patient. I never decided to move wards in the middle of the night. I never decided to watch that torturous scene unfold.

'I am never, ever going back there,' I whisper, looking up at the grey monstrosity of the hospital building looming against the London skyline as we make our way to the car.

'Never,' Finn nods, wrapping his arm around my shoulder.

The strange thing about touching death is that life resumes. On our way home, as I stare out of the car window, I'm struck by how the traffic lights still flash red, amber and green, pedestrians still walk into the road without looking, the morning trucks still pull up with deliveries for the local stores and people still sit chatting over steaming lattes in foggy cafe windows. The last 24 hours, for most people, won't be breaking news. 'Oh, she died in hospital,' they will think. 'She was very ill.' All the while, they're distancing the tragedy from their own lives, protecting themselves by putting it firmly in a box marked 'This wouldn't happen to me'. While you may be able to forget hearing a story about someone haemorrhaging to death in a hospital, you can never forget *seeing* it. I press my face against the window, watching the crowds pass by. I want to scream at the world to stop but the world stops for no one.

Over the next few months, my friends' lives continue to be occupied with happy chapters of love and laughter; pages filled with parties and hen-dos and weddings. They're currently living out their 'chick lit and romance' era. I try desperately to join them but my own chapters are something of a cross-genre that frequently spans 'horror' too. Our stories and their contents are entangled yet all vastly different; it's hard to tell what really goes on below their carefully crafted everyday façades. From the outside, everyone appears to be holding it together.

I shelve the story of the bowel haemorrhage for many years to come because part of me knows that is the only way to stop it from eroding all the pages that surround it. This way, if you don't look too closely, my own story can almost blend in with all of the others.

In the years that follow, the medics eventually decide that the reason I'm having repeated adrenal crises, and the reason my body seems to eat up the steroid meds like they're sweets, is that something *else* is putting my adrenal glands under pressure and requiring my body to need absurd amounts of cortisol. Eventually, after rounds and rounds of more investigations, it turns out the TB has *returned*. Thankfully, the medics confirm it isn't infectious.

All these years on, though, this illness still continues to haunt me, the 'great masquerader' parading in its many guises. I'm faced with the strange but familiar dichotomy of overwhelming relief that I, once again, have an explanation for how I'm feeling but also fear. Initially, when I hear the name 'TB', panic rushes through me as I visualise a future forever ensnared in the talons of this cruel disease. I allow myself some time to feel the raw emotion of it all, to acknowledge how frightening it is and to talk it through.

Afterwards, I do what I always do: brush myself down and focus only on the next step.

First time around, I wasted so much energy treading water behind the scenes, so desperate to avoid being seen as 'The Girl with TB'. This time, I decide to reframe the narrative; I remind myself that I am still here, persisting, despite it all. Instead of stigma, I try to see strength. I still don't discuss it in great detail but, from the outset, I do share the TB (take two) diagnosis with those around me, knowing that doing so will help them to understand. The illness may be the same but I'm determined that my approach is going to be different.

To ensure the TB goes once and for all, the medics now need to trial a new, stronger drug combination. For the first few weeks of treatment, I have to be supervised as a hospital inpatient. If this weren't all daunting enough, it happens to coincide with a global pandemic.

'You're so busy today,' I observe, as my nurse Reyna rushes from bed to bed.

'This is nothing,' she says. 'During the first lockdown, this was a Covid ward.'

'That must have been horrific.'

She nods.

'There were so many dying patients and not enough oxygen. During one of my shifts, a man died in that room over there.' She points across the corridor to a side room, opposite my bay. I want to tell Reyna to stop but it's clear that her dam has been filling up and up and today it has overflowed. She cannot stop, any more than I can stop her. 'I had to carry his dead body out of that room and swap him with a patient who was still alive and could maybe be saved with the oxygen.'

I want to reach over and hold her hand. Reyna is telling me about something so personal and yet, any human connection feels impossible to build. Social interaction relies on gesture, touch and expression, more things that have been stolen by this cruel virus. She hovers for a moment at the end of my bed, as if she wants to say more. I sense a desperate yearning for acknowledgement and yet the only person she has to offload onto is me, a patient, whose own dam is also on the brink of bursting. It seems we are all searching for a kind of acknowledgement. We are a nation flooded with nowhere to go.

My month in hospital during Covid-19, with no visitors, means my entire world becomes the patients on my ward. I already know more about these women than I do about people I've known my whole life. Some things are lovely to know: Olive has three granddaughters and gets this wistful glint in her eye whenever she talks about them. Some things I'd rather not know: Moira's stool was 'ginger' this morning. Some things make me sad: no one has dropped anything off for Sarita during the course of her three-week admission. Some things make me realise how lucky I am: Mum, Dad and Finn have dropped off little packages of food, drinks, cards and gifts every single day.

'My dad is going to the supermarket in a minute and wondered if any of you would like anything?' I say to my neighbours this afternoon.

'I'd like a newspaper please,' Moira says.

'Some orange juice for me please,' Olive says. 'I like the fresh one with the bits in.'

I already know Olive well enough to realise that standard concentrated orange juice will not suffice. She shows total disdain for every item on the hospital menu and her doting family only drop off luxury items from M&S.

'JAM DOUGHNUT!' I hear Sarita's voice boom from behind the curtain.

Sarita is from Spain and although I've attempted to resurrect a little of my Spanish vocab, she's mostly been too poorly to chat. She's always turned down the offer of any supplies.

An hour later, Dad obligingly rings the ward buzzer with our treats. I'm not allowed out of the bay but can visualise him at the entrance of the ward.

'From your father.' Today's nurse, Alexio, walks in, armed with our carrier bags.

Dad calls me from the car park. I can't see him but somehow it feels like we're closer that way. I begin rifling through the bags. Inside mine is a handwritten note from Mum explaining the contents. She's packed a homemade spread of containers filled with fresh salads, sandwiches, juices and cake. Alongside these are magazines, more cards from my friends and a gorgeous room spray from Finn. I really am one of the lucky ones.

I ask Alexio to hand out the goodies. The atmosphere is buzzing. Olive beams at her fresh organic juice and Moira dives into the newspaper. There is a pause while Alexio examines the jam doughnuts.

'Sarita, I'm really sorry but you're diabetic,' he says.

Sarita failed to mention this. I now have a vision of her collapsing as she tucks into the bag of pure sugar that I'm responsible for gifting her.

'*¡Es ridículo!* I look forward to jam doughnut all day.'

Talk about hopes raised and hopes dashed.

A few minutes later, Alexio re-enters our bay to check Sarita's blood pressure.

'GO AWAY!' Sarita shouts. 'You no let me have jam doughnut.'

The sad packet of doughnuts sits on my side table for the next three hours. Sarita has now fallen into a pit of despair. Alexio observes this and heads to my bedside.

'I've decided a jam doughnut will do Sarita good in other ways. So, I will give it to her, and I'll just give her some more insulin to counteract the sugar.'

My heart swells. Alexio has seen that this is so much more than a doughnut. This is an emotional boost to power Sarita through another day. He takes a doughnut out of the bag and takes it to her. I hear rustling behind the curtain.

'This is *lovely*! *Gracias*,' she calls over.

I smile but feel a twinge of sadness. Being in hospital during Covid is a lonely place to be. I can get through it because I know I am loved. I know there are people beyond the window – the window I can't walk up to or look out of – who are thinking of me, waiting for me and will be ready to give me the biggest hug when I get home. For the last three weeks, I have watched Sarita lie all alone in her bed; no one has dropped anything in and no one has called. Covid highlights a sad truth: our hospital wards are full of Saritas, patient upon patient with no one beyond the window.

After being discharged from hospital on the new TB drugs, I'm faced with that messed-up patient psychology of putting something into my body literally every single day that I know is making me feel horrific. The next 18 months are spent in a repetitive cycle of bed, sofa and freezing-cold showers. The drugs turn my skin red raw like my own body is setting fire to itself. Each morning, my skin is covered in actual burn marks and cuts where my own blood has boiled through the surface overnight. I figure if the meds are making me feel this toxic, they must be working. That's what keeps me going: the thought of a life *free* from this illness. However unbearable it gets, there's no way I'm missing a single dose. My new life is within touching distance and I will do whatever it takes.

'When the bluebells come it will be better,' Finn keeps reminding me, whenever I hit a low point.

I am due to finish my treatment in May. The bluebells have become my goal. These enchanting flowers hide away all year, then emerge in spring, colourful, flourishing and unstoppable. They have become my sign that I, too, will bloom again.

In my final week of treatment, at golden hour, Finn and I wander into the woods near Mum and Dad's house. We meander along a narrow path that opens up into an expansive forest glade. The soft hues of the evening sun float through the branches, illuminating a carpet of blossoming bluebells. Their clusters of delicate petals flicker in the dappled light, merging together like the flecks of an Impressionist painting.

Finn pulls a little pouch from his pocket and hands it to me.

'I was going to give this to you next week after you finished your treatment but I figure maybe you need it for the final push.'

From inside the pouch, I pull out a fine gold necklace. Gracefully hanging from the chain is a delicate bluebell. Finn moves my hair aside and places it around my neck. I hold the tiny bell between my fingers and look up at the hazy evening sky. I silently ask the universe that this is it: *In one week's time please make my life as a patient come to an end, forever.*

'When the bluebells come it will be better,' I whisper.

PATIENT SURVIVAL TIPS

- Death is always sad. Death is always traumatic. It is no better because it 'happened in a hospital'. Allow yourself time to feel and grieve.
- Say it out loud! Voicing your fears doesn't make them go away but it can make them feel that little bit less daunting than when they are endlessly spinning around in your head.
- A smile, a little chat or a small act of kindness can be enough to transform a fellow patient's entire day.
- Having a goal is everything. Never stop moving forwards.
- Find your sign!

17

HOPE

During the first few days after my TB treatment finishes, our flat increasingly resembles a florist. Every surface is bursting with bouquets sent from loving friends and family congratulating me on reaching the final hurdle. Tonight, to celebrate, Finn takes me out to my favourite little authentic Spanish restaurant at the end of our road. We drink sangria and eat paella by flickering candlelight.

'To your new life.' Finn raises his glass and his eyes glint with excitement for the future.

'To *our* new life.' I clink my glass to his, wanting this even more for Finn than I do for myself.

We spend the meal engaged in animated discussions, manifesting future holidays and socials. This evening, I take on the role of 'healthy Tilly', someone who can make plans, confident in the knowledge that she *will* be able to carry them out. I so badly want to trust that this is the moment we've been waiting for; but when I lie in bed and try to sleep at night, uncertainty creeps in. Will the meds' awful side effects subside? Will I no longer spend my nights in the freezing-cold shower? Will I stop spending my days in ice hats? Will adrenal crises be things of the past? Will I get some sort of normality?

It turns out the answer to all of these questions is no. Far from living my best life, over the next six weeks, life gets worse than I ever could have imagined. My body jumps into full-on attack mode. My muscles spasm and lock and visibly twitch. The pain in my flank contracts deep inside. My skin no longer burns only at night but also throughout the day. Finn regularly wanders into the bathroom to find me plunging my head under the cold bathwater or dousing my limbs with the freezing shower. My cheeks, lips and eyes randomly swell. My faces rages as though I'm suffering a reaction to an insect bite, but there's no trigger – just my own body stinging itself again and again. One morning, I notice a little scab on my ankle. With each day that passes, it spreads, coiling in circular red spirals like a venomous snake across my foot. It feels like poison building and penetrating through my skin, erupting in oozing pustules. I lose a stone in weight in six weeks but my tummy begins to grow. Then, all of my symptoms start to kick off at once in gruelling attacks. I have no idea what's causing them or how to calm them.

Once again, I begin the rounds of medics, desperately searching for an explanation. Nobody has one. Mum resumes her relentless research, putting a whole host of suggestions forward. No one will engage. 'You've come off the treatment now; things should be getting better,' the medics all say.

I trace my eyes over the abundance of cards lining our windowsills, the vibrant 'Congratulations!' 'You did it!' 'So proud of you!' now tormenting me. Everyone so badly wants me to be better. I so badly want to be better but my life has taught me that wanting something doesn't make it happen. Far from holidaying and socialising, Finn and I retreat to the sanctuary of my family home, mostly because we are scared. My body is being unpredictable. We're never sure what's coming next.

Tonight, I'm about to head downstairs. I go to place one leg in front of the other, an automatic action that I've never considered before. My brain is telling my leg to extend, telling my foot to press down onto the step in front of me, but it won't move. The muscles in my calves quiver and then ping, like a series of elastic bands snapping and becoming lax.

'I'm stuck,' I wail, as my legs buckle beneath me. I collapse onto the stairs.

Usually, I'm like a set of neat, colour-coded crayons, secured by a strong elastic band. To the outside world, I'm holding it together. Tonight, the band snaps and the crayons fling across the floor in a messy sprawl. Angry reds, lonely blues, simmering ambers, startling yellows and numb greys, a colour palette of different emotions, all competing for space among my irrepressible sobs.

Finn and Dad race to the bottom of the staircase. Mum runs down the landing behind me. They climb the steps and surround me, my own elastic bands, holding me tight, momentarily assembling me back together again.

'This can't go on. We need to get her into a hospital,' Mum whispers.

Mum is right. This sort of extreme bodily reaction should equal get yourself to hospital ASAP but her words are tinged with an unspoken fear. We've been trying to navigate getting me admitted for weeks now and it's proving impossible. None of us can contemplate that I can be this ill and be in this much pain and still be unable to access hospital care.

Over the last few years, I've mostly been admitted to hospital in adrenal crises. Having a named condition means there has been a protocol and pathway to follow, either through the GP or A&E. It certainly hasn't been easy to navigate. Rare conditions often aren't well understood and rely on a lot of self-advocacy; but in the past, having my Addison's label has at least got me through the hospital doors. The last few months have been different; this isn't an adrenal crisis. Instead, I've slowly deteriorated at home, with a plethora of unexplained symptoms affecting multiple systems in my body. We keep being told that I need to be dealt with as an outpatient, by a specialist who has the time to carry out the tests and uncover the diagnosis.

At each outpatient appointment, I'm asked the same question: 'So, what is your *primary* complaint?'

'My whole body,' I say truthfully, but I know this isn't the answer the doctors want to hear.

I can't say my 'headaches' or 'burning skin' or 'muscle spasms' or 'kidney pain' or 'digestion' or 'swellings' or 'weakness' or 'dizziness' or 'weight loss' are the *main* problem. One minute my headache is unbearable, the next I'm crying out with my vibrating muscles. Sometimes they all erupt simultaneously.

Each specialist is only interested in looking at their discipline. I imagine taking a photograph of my whole body and cutting it up into horizontal strips, separating all the different parts of me. The doctor holding the photo of my head has no idea what my feet look like. I am reduced to a series of body parts, all viewed in isolation. To solve my case, I need a holistic approach, where the medics collectively piece the photograph back together again. Instead, I am trapped in a system that relies on putting people in boxes. Bodies aren't made for boxes.

We are now lost in a barren landscape, with no signs or map to guide us. Every route we take ends in the same way; roadblock after roadblock forcing us to turn around.

Over the last few months, we've been told:

'You won't solve this on your own . . .'
'Your GP won't solve this . . .'
'There's no point going to A&E. They won't know what to do with you and won't have the resources to investigate this, so you'll just be discharged . . .'
'Even a billionaire wouldn't solve your case self-funded . . .'
'Without a named condition, we can't put you under a team in hospital yet . . .'

I'm dealing with a broken system. It won't accept me without a diagnosis but how is anyone with a rare condition ever meant to get a diagnosis? I always pride myself on being positive and believing it will work out; but after a series of futile appointments, as I sit on the stairs tonight, in the arms of Finn and my family, I can sense that even they don't have a plan. And without a plan, I'm frightened.

Mum keeps reiterating her mantra: 'Doing something is always better than doing nothing.' This morning, I hear her on the phone to

Nathan, the secretary of my Addison's consultant, Dr Bek. I smile as she asks how his son is getting on at his new school. Mum never just does a polite 'Hello'. She always asks about other people's lives and finds out their story.

'Dr Bek will see you tomorrow,' she exclaims at the end of the call, flinging her arms around me.

'Thanks to you and Nathan being best mates.' I lean into her, relief surging through me.

The next day, I struggle to walk into the appointment, my withering limbs now hardly able to hold up my skinny body. My face is barely visible behind the patchwork of pain plasters covering my skin. Underneath my eyes are deep purple crescents. I am unrecognisable.

I tell Dr Bek that I'm on 240mg of hydrocortisone steroid through the day and night. Most Addison's patients need 20mg and see serious weight gain if they up the dose just a tiny bit. I am rapidly fading away, at 48kg.

'The last doctor I saw felt the steroid must be helping to treat *another* condition. He told me to keep injecting until someone could get me admitted to hospital,' I explain.

'Well, I agree this certainly isn't an adrenal crisis,' Dr Bek says. 'But yes, it's possible the steroid is calming down inflammation related to a separate, undiagnosed condition.'

On the basis that Dr Bek doesn't feel this illness fits under endocrinology, he can't admit me under his team – but he does have a colleague who he thinks may be able to help.

'He's the master at solving rare, complicated cases,' Dr Bek says.

Relief overwhelms me. At last, in this barren landscape, there is a road sign ahead.

Dr Bek immediately picks up the phone to Professor Deacon, a senior professor at one of the London hospitals. By 9am the next day, I'm sitting in Professor Deacon's waiting room.

I look down at my legs and squirm. I remember all those years ago, outwardly gasping at a lady in the hospital cafe whose legs epitomised the description 'thin as twigs'. Now mine look the same. My muscles have wasted away, uncovering the sharp bone of my shins beneath. Mum gives me her arm as we enter the appointment. I place all my bodily weight onto it, allowing her momentum to guide me forward.

Professor Deacon takes one look at me.

'Do you not think you need to be *in* a hospital, Tilly?'

'Yes, yes I do,' I whisper.

Mum explains all the avenues we've tried to get me admitted. Hearing her say it out loud again makes me see it for what it really is: absurd.

'You need to lie down.' Professor Deacon gently guides me over to the bed at the side of his consulting room. He turns to Mum.

'She'll die if we leave her at home. She *needs* to be admitted *now*.' He picks up the phone on his desk. It seems Professor Deacon is senior enough to override the system. Finally, the roadblock has been lifted.

He walks towards the side of the bed.

'This has been a total fuck-up but I am going to get you better, Tilly.'

I take in the steely conviction in his eyes. I realise I believe him. This man wants to help me. Before we leave, he scrawls his name and number down on a piece of paper and hands it to Mum.

'Take her straight to A&E. They're expecting her. Call me if you have *any* problems.' He rushes outside into the corridor and returns with a wheelchair.

Mum attempts to take the chair from him but Professor Deacon insists on personally wheeling me all the way to the entrance of his clinic. Mum's eyes are now watery. We're not used to this.

'Thank you. Thank you. Thank you,' I say over and over again.

My words aren't enough to express the enormity of what Professor Deacon has offered me today. He has given me a lifeline.

I feel like I've entered a kind of parallel universe. From the moment I arrive in A&E, everything that Professor Deacon said would happen *happens*. I'm seen quickly. The doctors assure me I will definitely be admitted and that *loads* of tests have been ordered. In the evening, a friendly nurse called Blessing arrives to wheel me up to the ward.

'You're heading to the best ward in the entire hospital.'

This feels like a good start.

'And if you get Beds 14 to 19, then you'll have a panoramic view of the whole of London.'

Mum squeezes my shoulder.

'Oh, luxury, Tilly.'

When the nurse at the station on Ward 7 informs me that I'll be in Bed 19, I feel like I've won the lottery. I'm wheeled into a spotlessly clean bay of four. My bed is next to the outer wall, lined with tall glass panes. Just as Blessing promised, the London skyline glitters against the night sky. I can see the Shard, St Paul's and Big Ben from my bed. A full moon glows through the window, bathing my bay in a soft, silver hue. It envelops me and makes me feel safe.

'Now, we hear you've had a really traumatic few weeks, Tilly.' The ward sister, Jenny, is standing at the end of my bed. 'So, we thought maybe it would be nice if your mum stayed with you tonight, what do you think?'

I am speechless. I stare up at her, unable to wrap my head around it all.

'That's so kind,' I murmur. 'Yes please.'

Jenny glances at the hard plastic chair next to my bed, the sort of chair Mum has spent a lifetime sleeping (or more like *not* sleeping) in. She rushes off and emerges a few minutes later with a squishy turquoise armchair and a remote control that stretches it out into a bed.

'Hopefully this will be a bit comfier for you.'

She hands over a pillow and blanket and Mum stares up at her with the same astonished expression as mine. Usually, we struggle to get a pillow for *me*, let alone for Mum.

'Oh, Jenny, this is unbelievable. You've all been so lovely to us.'

'Just doing our job,' Jenny smiles.

The next morning, not one but *four* different teams of doctors come to see me. I'm so used to having to gabble my complex medical history out in five minutes flat on the morning ward round that

I find myself talking at a million miles per hour. I realise I can slow down. These doctors are different. They interject, ask questions, request that I expand and give more detail. They sit down next to my bed and write copious notes. They are receptive to Mum's endless years of research. They read her files of medical letters. They are fascinated by the photos of how my face swells and rash flares. They even ask to make copies to take to their meetings.

'Professor Deacon is a god,' is a line they each repeat.

It feels like they are all under instruction from this 'god' that they *must* solve my case. It feels weird, but good weird – like everyone is saying, 'Professor Deacon has got this. He's going to get you better.'

'He's ordered loads of tests, and I mean *loads*,' Dr Holmes tells me.

'We're so grateful,' Mum and I say over and over again to everyone we meet.

Neither of us can believe I am actually here. Only a few days ago, it seemed like the heavy double doors at the front of every hospital had been slammed in our faces.

On Saturday morning, a porter called Stuart arrives at the end of my bed to wheel me down for a test.

'On a Saturday?' I look up at him, confused. Either I've got the day wrong or Stuart hasn't realised it's the weekend.

He nods, seemingly unperturbed.

True to his word, I am sent for a specialist neural examination on a *Saturday*. This shows it's possible. This hospital knows that being ill can't be confined from Monday to Friday, nine until five. Being ill is not a choice.

When I arrive back on the ward, I overhear a consultant about to start her ward round with her team of medical students and junior doctors.

'It will be boring if I just do all the talking and you just write notes . . .' she tells them. I think of all the terrified juniors I've seen cowering behind their notepads over the years. 'Let's make this a learning experience. You ask the *patient* questions and you ask *me* questions.'

'Is this place actually real?' I whisper to Mum.

My mind aches trying to work out how I've landed here. Why does Professor Deacon, who until this week had never even met me, want to help me? How have we stumbled upon this hospital?

'I just can't work it out,' I say to Mum.

'I think he could see how poorly you are, Tilly, and how you've just been left.'

'But I've been poorly so many times and no one ever does this much to help me. It feels different here.'

'You don't need to work it out. Just keep thanking the universe that it's happened,' Mum says.

PATIENT SURVIVAL TIPS

- 'Are you better now?' can begin to feel like a pressure, especially when the answer is always no. Be honest with your loved ones about how you *really* feel.
- Secretaries are the gatekeepers: they book in the appointments and they have the power to rearrange the doctor's diary.

- Celebrate the staff that go above and beyond. It may be their 'job', but the *way* they do it can make or break your whole hospital stay.
- Prep a file with all your medical letters, test results and scans. It will save you and the medics so much time down the line.
- Doing *something* always feels better than doing *nothing*.

18

ATTACK

'It's going to get me,' I cry.

I know what's coming.

A wave of sweat flows down my back. A strong metallic scent radiates from me. I curl into a tight ball, clutching my agonising, boiling-hot head. My face begins to swell. The muscles in my calves visibly spasm. I grip my armpits, which rhythmically contract. Sharp, stabbing pains erupt through my flank. The rash on my foot rages, spirals of venomous snakes slithering across the surface of my skin, oozing pustules of yellow liquid.

'No, it's not, Tilly,' Finn responds.

Finn saw these attacks begin back at home but they hadn't yet reached these heights. So far, in hospital, they've mostly kicked off at night. Ever since that first night, the doctors and nurses have actively encouraged Mum to stay. This never happens. I'm trying not to think about why. Part of me hoped Finn would never witness the torturous scenes we've been dealing with since arriving here, but now the attacks are building, ravaging my body and ripping through my insides with lethal force night and day. This afternoon, Dad and Finn get a live viewing.

'You're not going to let it win, Tilly,' Finn says. 'You are going to *beat it*.'

This isn't stopping anytime soon. I know the pattern now. The sweat engulfs me. My hair is wet. My clothes are wet. The sheets are wet. I scream out as electricity courses through my veins, sparking, pulsing and then exploding through my muscles with uncontrollable force. It surges down my leg, rumbles through my calf and then fuses as it blasts my foot. My right foot drops, hanging from my ankle, stuck at a strange angle like it's disconnected from my body. In other moments, it flows down my fingers, pinging them upwards. My body has become a circuit with someone else pressing the buttons. My temperature rises. My blood pressure soars. My heart rate gets faster and faster. When it reaches 180, the monitors around my bed frantically flash and bleep.

'I think we need a doctor,' Mum calls to the nurse.

As brilliant as the doctors have been with their planned visits, asking to see them in an acute episode has proved more challenging. We've found that 'someone is having a heart attack' tends to beat 'someone is having a strange, painful-looking, atypical attack'. My own 'team', as I affectionately call them – Mum, Dad and Finn – usually end up having to come up with their own ways to get me through.

'Juice, apple juice,' I murmur.

'I'm addicted to apple juice,' said no one ever. And yet, in every attack my body demands that I fill it with litres upon litres of it. I'm also an addict with very particular taste; my body demands that only the *cloudy* variety will do. The rate I'm now knocking these back is displaying a *need*, rather than a want. I'm certain it's doing something to save me.

'You've always known your own body. Listen to what it's telling you,' Mum says, whenever I question this bizarre ritual.

We now have a stash of cloudy Pink Lady apple juice at the ready. Our own bedside pharmacy.

Dad leans into my side cupboard and pulls out a bottle. He places a paper straw into it and scoops my head forward to hold it to my lips. I slurp it back. Then reach for another.

'Ice? Could we try ice to cool her down?' Finn asks, watching the beads of sweat trickle down my forehead.

'Good plan.' Dad races off to search some out.

'Focus on your breathing, Tilly,' Mum tells me.

She stands at the end of my bed, motioning for me to slow my fast and shallow breaths. A few minutes later, Dad emerges holding a plastic cup from the ward kitchen. He drips the cubes onto my head, cooling down the fire burning within. Finn perches on the edge of my mattress and begins to rub essential oils into my vibrating calves.

It is a scene of love among a scene of torture.

'How about we *show* them, Tilly?' Mum says, pointing to her phone.

'Yes, film, film.' The pain takes over again, enveloping my body in its wrath. I return to my ball, writhing in silent agony.

'I hate having to do this.' Mum hovers above me, filming the brutal attack on her phone.

We assumed that when an attack started we'd be able to press my call-bell and a doctor would emerge. The reality is they usually arrive an hour later, when the attack has already ended. This clip is going to be a real-life horror movie to watch back but it could change things. Now we'll be able to show all the doctors who visit my bedside what the attacks look like. Seeing is different to hearing.

Today's attack lasts so long that when Dr Sims arrives, she doesn't have to observe it through Mum's screen. An hour in, the live viewing continues in front of her eyes.

'Now, this doesn't look like somewhere anyone would choose to be,' I hear her say. Her voice is gentle. She takes my stats, notes down my vital signs and orders more pain relief but she's helpless to stop the attack. 'We need to find the cause,' I hear her say. 'Until then, we can only try to manage the symptoms.'

'The attacks are dreadful,' Dad says.

'We always say it's good when the tests come back "normal", but in this case maybe not,' Dr Sims says.

She's right. 'Normal' doesn't help when you know something seriously *abnormal* is happening to your body.

'What would you like to do, Tilly, when you're better?' she asks. Dr Sims tries to help me escape to a world beyond the hospital curtain but I'm in too much pain to answer.

'Tilly would love to be active,' Mum says.

My flank crunches. It feels like my kidneys are trying to excrete a deadly poison.

'What would you like to do, Tilly?' Dr Sims asks.

Survival mode leaves no room for conversation.

'She'd like to be up a mountain,' Finn says.

Dr Sims starts to describe a scene of a snow-capped mountain glistening in the winter sun. That's where I'd like to be.

'What else would you like to do, Tilly?'

'She loves to write,' Mum says.

'She wants to write a book one day,' Finn says.

'I'll look forward to reading it, Tilly,' Dr Sims says.

For over half an hour, as the attack continues, she keeps observing me, talking to me and encouraging me, even though I can't reply. She tries to help me visualise a future beyond these walls. Dr Sims takes the time to see what is right in front of her, the girl I really am, the girl I want to be.

I scream out again as a new wave of venom floods my veins. I've been poorly before but what this illness is doing to my body is inhumane. No human should have to go through it. No human should have to see it. This attack lasts over an hour and a half. It is relentless.

I know it's coming to an end when I have a sudden, desperate urge to urinate. This has become the pattern. Each attack ends with a vast, unnatural volume of urine. Afterwards, I sink onto my back, gasping for breath.

'It's like you've run a marathon,' Dr Sims comments.

I look up, taking in her brown bob and kind eyes for the very first time.

'Am I going to die?' I whisper.

She doesn't answer.

A week on, my second attack of the day has just come to an end. Still, no one has any clue what they are or why they're happening. I've now had bloods, neural examinations, ultrasounds, urine tests and even a full-body PET scan – more tests than anyone has ever done on me before – but still no diagnosis.

'What if I never get better?' I whisper to Mum.

This evening, beyond my window, the candyfloss clouds float against the London horizon. I feel tiny and insignificant up here, thinking of all the lives and stories unfolding across the vast and sprawling city below.

'You will,' Mum says. 'What was it Dr Holmes said earlier?' She looks over at me.

'The "best medical brains in London" are searching for this,' I recount.

'You've certainly never had that before. I know it's really hard, Tilly, but that's what you have to hold onto.'

A muffled cry erupts from the other side of my curtain, then another dry squawk, followed by a rapid succession of gasping, heaving breaths. The call-bell flashes above my neighbour's bed. Mum glances around the ward.

'Handover,' she says, turning her phone to face me, illuminating the time.

We are now expert enough to know that 8pm means the nurses on the day shift will be handing over to the night shift, giving the new team an update on all the patients on the ward. Great in theory, but not so great if at 8pm your meds are due, or at 8pm you're bursting for the toilet, or at 8pm you descend into a life-threatening medical emergency and *every* member of staff is tied up in a team meeting.

The cacophony continues. Mum leaps from her chair and pokes her head into next door's cubicle. The cries increase in volume.

'Oh, you poor love,' I hear Mum exclaim. 'I'll get someone right now.'

A few seconds later, footsteps rush into our bay.

'I don't think she can breathe,' Mum says.

'I'll get a doctor now,' I hear Sister Jenny respond.

For the next 30 minutes, our bay is chaotic as doctors and nurses race in and out of my neighbour's cubicle holding tubes and bags. The gasps subside and give way to a medley of muffled conversations, concise instructions and caring words of reassurance. When a sense of calm is finally restored, a doctor I've never seen before pokes her head through my curtain.

'I just wanted to thank you,' she says, looking at Mum. 'You saved a life today.'

Late at night, when the lights have been turned off and we are just about to attempt to try to sleep, my neighbour appears at the end of my bed. She's middle-aged, wearing a starchy jay-cloth hospital gown and holding a large plastic cylinder full of translucent watery blood, attached to her body through a long thin tube.

'I couldn't sleep before I thanked you for what you did for me today,' she says to Mum.

'Don't be silly, I'm just glad I was here.'

'My lung bag had completely filled with fluid.' She gestures to another bag hanging underneath her gown. 'It needed emptying and was backflowing up, so I was suffocating.'

'You must have been terrified,' Mum says.

'It would happen at handover, wouldn't it?' The lady rolls her eyes. 'I work as a ward manager at a different hospital. When I first joined, they also had every member of staff doing the handover at the same time. It was one of the first systems I changed.'

'Good for you,' I say. 'It makes no sense.'

'There's not much point in *handing over* a patient who's dead,' she laughs. 'I'm Abebi, by the way.'

Abebi goes on to tell us that she finished cancer treatment last year. The cancer has now gone but since, fluid keeps collecting in her tissues and getting infected.

'I'm so sorry, I've been the world's worst hospital roomie,' I say. 'I've probably kept you awake all night, having these awful attacks.'

'Never be sorry. I'm just so sad to hear you suffering.'

'They still don't know what's causing them,' Mum says.

Abebi now looks me directly in the eyes.

'I can tell that your mind is very strong, Tilly; and because of your mind, your body is going to get better.'

Tonight, as I attempt to sleep, my new friend's words reverberate through me and fill me with a little confidence that there are more chapters in my story.

Over the next week, my attacks become so frequent that more doctors are given a live viewing. I try to tell myself this is a good thing. This is how my case will be solved. Another part of me is frightened. The attacks are also becoming more brutal. It feels like I'm running out of time.

This morning, my body dramatically deteriorates when my Addison's consultant, Dr Bek, happens to be doing his ward round.

'The teams are running out of ideas,' he says.

This is not what I want to hear.

'Obviously I'm not a doctor . . .' Mum begins. 'But as a very desperate mother, I have been researching. This seems to be something that gives chronic symptoms, with acute attacks, and it appears to respond to sugar. We've noticed the attacks calm a little if she glugs back apple juice when she feels them coming on. Are there any conditions that could present like this?' Mum asks.

Dr Bek thinks for a moment.

'I do have one idea,' he says, as I recoil into my ball, clutching my quivering calves. My abdomen seizes like it's been locked in a vice. Electricity surges through me, blasting with a force so strong my whole body convulses. I cry out in excruciating pain. *Ideas. Yes please. We need ideas.*

'I wonder if this could be porphyria,' he hypothesises.

Porphyria. Porphyria. Porphyria. In the haze of the attack, the word swirls around my head. It's a word I'm already familiar with. 'Porphyria's Lover' was the poem I cited as igniting my love of English Literature in my Oxford Uni interview. Where most applicants were probably singing the praises of Keats's Romantic verses, I opted to discuss Robert Browning's poem about a dark and haunting murder by strangulation. Perhaps slightly concerning aged 17, but whatever floats your boat. It got me in.

Dr Bek assures us he'll look into it. After he leaves, Mum flicks up her research list of 'possible diagnoses' in the notes on her phone. She hovers her finger over the word 'Porphyria'.

'We've discussed this one, Tilly. Porphyria is a condition where poisonous "porphyrins" build up in the bloodstream. It's the test where the blood and urine can't be exposed to light,' Mum tells me, clicking on the link to the report she already had saved. 'One of the treatments is glucose.'

The more Mum reads, the weirder it seems.

'You have all the symptoms,' she says.

The poem. Mum's list. The juice. It all feels like the universe is trying to give us a sign.

A few hours later, we're in the basement of the hospital, waiting for a porter to wheel me back up to the ward after another scan. My face begins to twitch. The metallic smell radiates from me. My legs start to vibrate.

'Oh no, it's starting.'

This will be my fourth attack of the day. The most I've ever had.

Mum asks if she can wheel me back up to the ward.

'I'm afraid we're not allowed to let you,' the secretary at the desk says. 'In case anything was to happen to her.'

Minutes later, my limbs begin to jerk. The secretary looks over at me. He wavers for a few seconds, then jumps from his seat.

'I *used* to be a porter . . .' He pauses, as I begin to shake. 'Yep, I'll just take her.'

Hooray for John the secretary and his logical loophole that means I make it back to the ward in time for the full-on convulsion to begin. Well, that's what I think. What actually happens is there's a glucose drip at the side of my bed – a glucose drip that is going to change everything.

Within moments of this drip full of sugar flooding my veins, my seizing, spasming muscles begin to calm. My withering body feels like it's coming back to life again. I don't descend into the full-on convulsion. Glucose treats porphyria. Surely this is evidence.

A nurse comes over and asks me to provide a sample.

'Is it OK to do while she's on this drip?' Mum asks. 'As I think the glucose is maybe a treatment.'

'Yep, fine.'

'I think the test also has to be done in the dark,' Mum says.

'Maybe put some tissue around it,' she responds.

I glance up at Mum. If the sample bag is opened, the tissue will just fall off, exposing the test to light. Tissue also isn't opaque. This test could change my life. We have to do it properly.

Cue Mum heading off on a casual life-or-death trip to the supermarket to purchase tin foil. Upon her return, we both head into the toilet and switch off the light. Peeing in those sample pots is an art I've perfected over the years. I now pride myself on having impeccable aim but peeing without being able to *see* the pot, with a body that is vibrating and a bladder that keeps contracting, is a whole different ball game. My entire hand and arm are now covered in urine. Mum labels the pot and wraps it in layers of tin foil. It's ready to go.

We're told the test needs to be taken to a dark room before it closes. It has to arrive quickly, as a special technician is waiting for it, and then it needs to be sent urgently to a specialist unit at another hospital, otherwise it will be left in the lab over the weekend. It's now Friday afternoon. The problem is there's now no one available to take it.

Yaz, one of the healthcare assistants, is just about to go on her break.

'Please, please can you find someone to take this? My daughter's life could depend on it,' Mum says to her.

She hovers for a few seconds, then puts down her coffee and turns to Mum.

'Come with me.'

Yaz proves to be my hero of the day. Running from Floor 9 to the basement, to avoid the world's slowest lift system, she gets my sample to the lab before it closes.

While we await my porphyria result, I'm told I'm going to be moved into a side room. It seems the horror show has now become too terrifying for public viewing. The thought of my own room would usually be absolute hospital goals but this move now means saying goodbye to my new friend Abebi. I've started to cherish the moments where Abebi pulls up a chair and shares stories of the ward she manages or shows me photos of her children or describes her Nigerian customs and culture. In turn, by asking about my own life, she occasionally allows me to glimpse Tilly, the girl beyond the patient, the one I am fighting to bring back. Now, when Finn arrives at the hospital armed with fresh juices for me each day, he always makes one for Abebi too.

'Thank you, Finn. And thank you, universe,' she says, as he hands over today's delicacy of carrot, apple and celery.

We bond over our joint catchphrase, grateful for any moment the universe gives us a break. On day one, Abebi was a complete stranger. Over the last week, with just a thin curtain between us, I've had no choice but to let her in. She's now seen me at my most vulnerable, heard me utter thoughts I would never verbalise to even my closest friends and witnessed scenes I would hate for them to ever glimpse. Abebi has crossed the boundary into the 'patient' part of my life, normally reserved for my team and my team alone.

Over the last few weeks, my friends have tried so hard to be there for me; my phone is filling with messages but I don't know what to say to them. Liv and Sammi have kept dropping off fresh coffees at the ward on their way to work. Phoebe and Eve have rocked up unannounced with baked goods. Only yesterday, my friend Rachel, who I've known since nursery, arrived with a selection of homemade salads and chocolate brownies. She printed a pretty menu to go alongside them, turning 'meals on wheels' into a moment to savour. Dad has always described Rachel and me as 'two peas in a pod' but my pod feels separate now. I've refused to let her or anyone else see me. My friends belong to a different world; how can they possibly relate?

When Abebi says, 'I know how you feel,' she really *does* know how I feel. I open up to her in a way that catches me off guard. It's like there's a magnetic energy connecting us, two people thrown together through suffering, united by adversity. She appeared just when I needed her.

Before we leave the ward, Abebi hands me a paper napkin with her number scrawled on the front.

'You must message me when you get your diagnosis and get better.'

As the nurse wheels me out of the bay and I make my journey to my new room, I visualise doing just that.

*

'Room' doesn't feel like a fair description for what we enter next. 'Luxury penthouse apartment' would be more appropriate. One entire wall is made of glass panes, showcasing a panoramic view of London. All we need are a few cocktails and overpriced nibbles and we could easily be at the top of the Shard.

'Want to know a secret?' Nurse Lucia says. 'For the private ward directly below, patients pay hundreds a night for this *exact* room. That's just for the room, no tests included . . . the only difference is their food is served on a silver tray.'

I take in my wooden desk, ensuite bathroom and the famous stretch of London attractions I can spot from my bed. There's even a guest bed folded up in the corner.

'We'll have to get you a silver tray then, Tilly,' Dad laughs.

As golden hour comes around, the view from my window becomes even more mesmerising. The sun dips down towards the horizon, bathing the sky in a buttery warmth. Its orange hues melt through the tapestry of glass, metal and stone, turning the London landmarks into silhouettes against the evening sky. They hold my gaze in a trance.

The moment is interrupted by a knock at my door. I keep staring ahead, waiting as long as possible, knowing that a quick blink is all it will take for my mind to jump back to the darker reality of life within these walls.

A doctor I've never seen before stands in the doorway.

'I've come to discuss your porphyria test.'

With the attacks deteriorating by the day, the doctors are now administering the glucose drip more regularly. Each time it enters my blood stream, it's like nectar to a bee. When it's removed, I quickly descend into an attack. Mum has now focused all her research on porphyria and similar conditions. The more she learns, the more it fits. It feels like everything rests on this test.

'We need to ask you to redo the sample,' the doctor says.

It turns out that, despite all our efforts with the tin foil, the sample was exposed to light somewhere later in the process and the test is flawed. I want to scream but instead smile politely and thank him for informing me.

Today I am consumed with an emptiness, hollowing me out from my core. Right now, I am meant to be walking up the aisle as a bridesmaid at our friends' Bella and Josh's wedding. Instead, Finn and I are still stuck in hospital.

'How about I read you some of their messages?' Finn suggests this evening.

I stare ahead, ignoring him.

'I think it would be good for you.' He picks up my phone. 'What do you think?'

I think my life chapters can be firmly described as 'horror' now, totally alienated from the summer romance my friends are currently cruising through. We exist in totally separate worlds. Their happy words don't belong here. Finn looks so eager, though, so desperate to do something to lift me.

'OK,' I say, for him more than for me.

He picks up my phone and reads me a message Bella sent this morning.

Today won't be the same without you Tilly but I promise, we will have a wedding Take Two when you're better.

'But I'm not getting better,' I say to Finn.

He scrolls through my phone again.

'This might cheer you up.'

He proceeds to read out a message from my friend Nina, asking if she can visit tonight, before she moves to Norway tomorrow. I've lost all sense of time in here. I had no idea Nina's move had already come around. This news from the world beyond my window jolts me.

'Would you like to see her?' Finn asks.

I lie flat on my back, staring up at the ceiling, gripping my yellow cushion to my tummy. It has now locked so hard, I can't physically move. Deep purple bruises litter my skin, cannulas hang from my hands and arms and my face is barely visible under the layers of anaesthetic pain patches covering my cheeks and forehead. I don't want anyone to see me like this but I suddenly have this sinking feeling that I must see Nina.

What if? What if . . .? I don't actually let myself say the words, but I just know I must see her before she leaves.

Later this evening, Nina appears in my doorway. The second her eyes fall on me, she bursts into tears.

'Not great for my self-confidence.' I muster a smile.

'I'm only crying because I'm so happy to see you,' she says.

For the next hour, Nina describes all the fun things we're going to do when I visit her in Norway when I'm better; from swimming in the fjords, to visiting the Royal Palace and hiking up mountains.

We reminisce about childhood holidays spent together at her *bestemor*'s (grandmother's) house.

'*Jeg elsker deg* [I love you],' I say to her, in my best Norwegian, before she leaves.

She sits beside my bed and holds my hand.

'Remember, you are the dandelion, Tilly.'

I smile.

'And dandelions don't just thrive in lush green fields . . .' she begins, then places her hand out for me to continue.

'But also in rough cracks between the pavement,' I finish.

PATIENT SURVIVAL TIPS

- *Showing* can be more powerful than *telling*. Document any visible symptoms with photos and videos.
- Research, research, research. You can only ask the next question if you have the knowledge to back up what you're saying.
- One test could change your life. Make sure it's done under all the correct conditions.
- Someone out there will really *get* what you're going through and you may find them in the most unexpected ways.
- Let the outside in.

19

HELL

I may have the worst luck medically but when it comes to my team, I am one of the luckiest. Dad and Finn work full time and yet there hasn't been a single evening that they haven't made the four-hour round trip from home to see me. Some nights they glimpse me for only a fleeting five minutes before I descend into an attack or visiting hours are over. They say it doesn't matter; they feel closer this way. It's Mum, though, who is my constant, with me night and day.

When a flamingo mother raises her chick, she loses her beautiful pink colour; a visible manifestation of the way she is transferring her own energy into her young. Once her little one is thriving, the flamingo mother regains her pink colour. The problem is that, all these years on, I'm still not thriving. Mum has spent a lifetime trying to give me any 'pink' moments she possibly can. It makes me so sad seeing the way this horrible illness is, once again, sapping her own colour, but she always tells me that she could never embrace life knowing I was suffering.

'I wouldn't be pink at all,' she says.

Now, after three weeks caring for me, while also operating a

24/7 medical research hub at my bedside, we can all see that Mum is fading. Thankfully, flamingos live in a 'flamboyance' and so do we. We have so many special people in our lives constantly offering to help and there is no one more willing than Mum's sister, Auntie.

'Support services!' Auntie grins, bustling into my hospital room this evening.

I adore Auntie, I trust Auntie and we can all 100 per cent rely on Auntie. She's the fifth member of our team, the only other person I'll let see it all. Tonight, she's driven five hours down the motorway from Manchester to be with us.

'I'm not quite Professor Rose . . .' She embraces Mum in a long, warm hug. 'But I make a pretty good deputy.'

'I can see the writing on the wall. Now that Auntie's rocked up, they'll no doubt diagnose you and start treatment and she'll wonder what all the fuss was about,' Mum laughs, leaning into Auntie's shoulder.

I close my eyes and let their chatter float over me. Mum's right, it will all be OK now that Auntie is here.

This evening, Mum leaves the hospital for a much-needed rest. A few hours later, a nurse pokes her head through my doorway.

'The drips seem to have helped a bit, so you don't need the side room anymore. You're off to Ward 6, AMU.'

Heading to AMU feels like a backward step.

'Dr Bek said that if I feel an attack coming on I have to ask for a bolus of steroid and for the glucose drip to restart. Can I just check these will definitely be written up on my new ward?' I ask.

'Of course.' She nods.

Auntie begins to pack up my room, loading my bed with our bags and emptying my windowsill of the cards from my friends. Moments later, a porter arrives.

By the time I reach my new bay, I feel that familiar wave of sweat seep from my skin. My tummy clenches like it's trapped in a brace. A series of electrical currents spark down my arms and legs.

'Oh no.' I glance up at Auntie. 'I need the drips.'

She nods, immediately pressing my call-bell. We wait and we wait and we wait. Nobody comes. Auntie goes up to the nurses' station. Ten minutes later, she returns on her own.

'There's no one there.'

We keep pressing my bell. Eventually, a nurse appears at the end of my bed.

'Can I please have the steroid and glucose drips?' I ask.

'I'd need a doctor to sanction that,' she says.

'They already have.' I look towards Auntie. 'I'm meant to be able to ask for them on request.'

'Nothing here. I can't give them to you without a doctor sanctioning it.'

Pulses of electricity fire through my limbs. I know I have to speak through the pain. This nurse has to understand that I *need* these drips. The glucose drip has helped to calm my attacks and with my body under such abnormal levels of stress and pain, I am still requiring high-dose steroids to control my Addison's disease.

Auntie sees me struggling and steps in, calmly reading from her notepad where she's logged the exact dosages and instructions from

Dr Bek, as well as the precise time I last had them. The nurse says she'll look into it.

I hold my head, rocking gently from side to side, tracing my eyes along the repetitive creases of the blue curtain. In front of me, it begins to morph into a vast blue ocean, the crests of the waves rising and falling in rhythmical beats, before rolling in neat lines towards the shore.

'Tilly, Tilly . . .' A voice. A person in the ocean. Auntie.

'Yes?' I look up at her.

'What are you doing, sweetheart?'

'Nothing,' I murmur. The sea disappears. A crinkly blue hospital curtain encloses me in a cramped blue box. My finger pings upwards, my leg jerks, my cheek twitches. My breathing becomes fast and shallow. Pain sears through me. *Glucose. Steroid. I need the glucose and steroid.*

'Where are the drips?' My eyes dart frantically around the blue box. Without them I'm going to drown. The waves are now thrashing towards me, threatening to sweep me away. It's getting darker. Colourful lights dance across the inky sky. I stretch my arms high into the air, trying to reach up and grab the wavy streaks of green and yellow and red. They're too fast. They keep escaping me.

'Tilly, Tilly . . . What are you doing?'

Someone's calling my name. A hand clutches my shoulder. *Glucose. Steroid.* No, they're not giving me them. They're pushing me under. I need to get them. I need to keep swimming. I push the hand away.

'I don't know what to do. She's acting really strangely. Something isn't right.' The colourful beams give way to a thin strip light above my bed, illuminating the silhouette of Auntie in the chair beside me. 'I'm just onto your mum, darling. I'm a bit worried about you. Can you tell me what's happening?'

I stare at her. Lots of things are happening.

'I'm going to put you on speaker . . .'

Mum is now in the ocean with us. We're treading water together.

'I need the glucose. I need the steroid,' I say. Yes, that's what I need.

'She's right. She does need them. Can you ask the nurse again?' Mum's voice.

'Tilly's not making much sense. The nurse keeps telling me she's confused.'

'No, she's not confused about this. We were clearly told by Dr Bek that when an attack began she *had* to have the drips. They've been giving them to her all week on the other ward.'

Jellyfish. That's what the colours are. Jellyfish. The sea is awash with monsters. There are too many to avoid. Their tentacles brush against me without warning, stinging my arm, then my leg, then my tummy.

'What's happening to her?'

'Sheets are wet with sweat . . . wet hair . . . vibrating . . . limbs jerking . . . crying out . . . clutching head . . . rash . . . foot burning . . . yellow pustules . . . she's not making sense. I think you need to come.'

'Something's clearly changed since the drips were removed. Whatever happens, keep reiterating that there must be an *organic* cause for this.'

They keep talking and talking and meanwhile we're going to drown. The dark sea is closing in, cloaking us in its murky shadows. It crashes and roars and hisses. The noise thunders through my ears. I hold my hands tightly against them trying to block it out.

'Does she have any meds on her?' A nurse stands at the end of my bed.

'I'll check the bags. I think just her emergency steroid injection,' Auntie says. 'Have you asked a doctor about the steroid and glucose drip?'

'Yes, I've asked. I'll let you know if I hear anything.'

'She's acting a bit . . . strangely. I really think she does need those drips.'

'I've asked. I'll be back in a second to lock her meds in there.' The nurse points to a square white cupboard attached to the wall. On the front is a lock.

Auntie begins digging around in the bag at her feet. My eyes fall on the black box at the table on the end of my bed. My steroid injection box. *Think, Tilly. Think.*

'Toilet,' I mouth to Auntie.

She nods.

My weak, wobbly legs are shaky on dry land. Auntie stands up, holding my arm. With my other hand, in a swift and quiet motion, I clasp the black box, tucking it by my side. Auntie can't see this. She'll give it to the nurse. The nurse will take it away from me. Then I will die.

'Do you want me to come in with you?'

I shake my head.

The yellow moon beams above, so bright it blinds me. I sit down and unzip the black box. Inside are my vials of steroid and my needles. My life ring. I scan the horizon. Sink. Shower. Bin. I need to bury the black box at the bottom of the ocean where no one is going to find it. *Think, Tilly.* Sink. Shower. Bin.

'Tilly, are you OK? Tilly, can you unlock the door? Tilly?'

Knocks. Voices. I need to be quick.

I press my foot on the pedal at the base of the rectangular bin. The inside is lined with a reef of poisonous coral, swaying in yellow and black stripes. I take a breath and slip my hand in among it, my black box camouflaged in the crevice of the rocks. I spot a gown on the floor. I throw that on top. Then I rip some paper towels and let them float over my black box. I shut the lid.

'She must have it in there with her . . . Tilly, Tilly, can you open the door?'

I undo the latch. Auntie steps in.

'Where's your steroid box, Tilly?'

'I hear she's been hiding medication . . . the nurse said her auntie found it in the bin.'

'Something's really not right.' Mum has joined us in the sea. 'She's only started acting like this since the steroid and glucose have been withdrawn. She's meant to be written up for them PRN – whenever she needs them.'

'It seems like she's experiencing psychosis,' a man in a maroon wetsuit says.

The nurse locked my life ring in the treasure trove on the wall and threw away the key. She buried it deep into the sand, so I can't find it.

'Have you eliminated an organic cause?' Mum's voice.

'I'm just a junior doctor,' Maroon Wetsuit says. 'There's nothing in the notes about the drips.'

'She's in a lot of pain and will need more steroid, otherwise she could go into an adrenal crisis.' Mum's voice.

'It's the middle of the night. We'll have to wait until the morning when the consultants are in.' Maroon Wetsuit.

'She's really deteriorating. I think someone needs to do something now.'

Maroon Wetsuit swims right up to my face.

'Can you try to get some sleep now do you think, Tilly?'

I know he's trying to trick me. I can't sleep. If I sleep, I die. I need to find the steroid and I need to find the glucose. The waves crash above my head. I will them to keep coming, hoping they'll shake the treasure chest so hard it bursts open. Maroon Wetsuit drifts away in the current. I recoil away from the inky ocean, comforted by the safety of my life raft. It feels solid, reassuring and yet, I know it is the vessel that will carry me to death. If I stay here, I'll waste away, without my vital supplies. I have to be brave. I have to make my escape while I still have the strength.

Instinctively, I jump from my life raft and swim, faster than ever before, my arms pushing back the water, my legs thrashing. They all try to catch me. Maroon wetsuits, blue wetsuits, grey wetsuits. Mum. Auntie. Dad. Finn. I need to find the treasure.

In front of me, bobbing on the top of the sea, is a bottle of Coke. Glucose. A life ring to cling onto. I lean forward and grab it, pouring it down my throat. It's warm, no longer fizzy. It must have been in the sea for a long time waiting for me.

'Stop drinking that. Stop!' Blue Wetsuit calls.

I glug it back. The sugar refuels me, igniting my limbs to keep powering on. I spot a piece of wood clinging to the shore. A new life raft in the distance. I race forward.

'Stop that right now! You cannot rip the posters off the wall!' Blue Wetsuit throws herself over me, pinning me in the sand. I'm suffocating. I need to reach the surface for air.

I'm on a new boat now. This one has been steered into an oppressive, dark cave. At the mouth of the cave, the only route out, sits a grey swimmer. They've trapped me in this cave and placed a guard at the entrance. I am a prisoner of the sea. The jagged stones loom down on me, knives ready to attack. My eyes desperately search for an alternative escape route but each twisting passage ends in danger. My lip quivers, my eyes fill. I can feel the life being sucked from my core, my energy submerged in the currents of the vast ocean beyond. I am alone and I am scared. No one is going to find me here.

'You've been very bad, causing a lot of problems. You're not escaping now. We're watching you.' Blue Wetsuit.

I pull away, shielding my body with my arms. Her words push me deeper into the cave. My breathing erupts in shallow gasps.

'Do you have any meds on you?' she asks.

Meds. What does she mean? I squeeze my eyes shut, hold my hands to my ears. I wrap my arms around my legs, pulling them close to my chest, recoiling from the world. *Think, Tilly. Think.* What's happened? The treasure. The Coke. The poster. I open my eyes.

'Hello, did you not hear me?' She's a nurse, with blonde hair.

I'm no longer in a cave. I'm in a sterile bay of four. I'm in hospital. I shake my head.

'If you're lying, I'll find them.'

The boat. The waves. The treasure. I think maybe my mind isn't working properly. *Steroid. Glucose.* The messages are all jumbled. *Waves. Oceans.* Stop. Rational Tilly. Rational Tilly. I still need the steroid. I still need the glucose. This I know. Without them, I will die. I look down. Mum's handbag is beside me. How can Mum's bag be here when she hasn't been here? None of my team are here. They've all abandoned me. I start to cry.

Then, out of the corner of my eye, at the bottom of Mum's handbag, I spot two small bottles of apple juice. I smile through my tears. I knew Mum would never abandon me. She's sent a survival package out to sea to save me. Rational Tilly. I need more glucose. I lean down and pick up the juices, placing them beside me on the bed. I guzzle one bottle back. *Glucose. Tick.*

After this night at sea, my body is freezing cold and clammy, my arms are shaking, my flank stabs, I'm seasick, dizzy. Rational Tilly. I have Addison's disease. I'll need more cortisol to survive. I now need my emergency steroid injection. *Think.* Mum always carries a spare emergency steroid injection. I glance around the ward to check Blonde Nurse isn't watching. The guard on the chair is looking the other way. I delve into Mum's bag again. I spot the little pink case she always keeps it in. A tear spills down my cheek. Mum has saved me again. I slip the injection case under the sheet.

I'm bursting for a wee. The attacks. This is how they end. My bladder fills and fills, like it's trying to excrete a poison. I can see the toilet from my bed but if I ask to go, the guard will follow and Blonde Nurse will confiscate my injection. The risk is too great. I know what I have to do. *Pretend you're in the sea.* I close my eyes and let it out. The sheets soak around me. Survival isn't pretty.

Blonde Nurse returns.

'Bag search time. If you've lied to me and have any meds in here, I'll find them.'

She begins digging around in Mum's bag and then in my bag. I hold my breath, moving the pink case containing my injection underneath my thigh.

'Gross, your sheets are wet. Did you wet yourself?' she asks.

I'm so scared of her. I want Mum and Dad and Finn and Auntie. Where are they? Why have they left me?

'I'll be back in a minute to change your sheets and I suppose we better get you out of those wet clothes.'

I inhale. My heart is racing so fast it feels like it will rip my chest open. She's going to find my steroid injection. I glance up at the guard on the chair. She's busy on her phone. I know I'm drifting in and out. I'm Tilly in hospital. Then I'm in the sea. What's happening to me? I'm so dizzy, everything is becoming blurry. My head fills with immense pressure. Beads of sweat roll down my legs. I retch and retch. Then, I start to shiver. Rational Tilly. I know what I have to do. I have to stop an adrenal crisis. Feeling my way, I clasp the top of the glass vial in the sheet and pop it open. I balance the vial of steroid in the gap between my thighs, then tear open the pack containing the needle. I create a little space between my legs and the sheet, then position the needle downwards and pull the liquid up into the syringe. *You can do it, Tilly.* I close my eyes, take a deep breath in and dart the needle deep into my thigh muscle. Two minutes. You're meant to inject it over two minutes. Blonde Nurse moves past the glass screen. I hold my breath. She's always watching me.

'New sheets.' She throws her net, ready to ensnare me.

I clench my teeth and press my jaws together as the steroid blazes down my leg. If I move or cry out, she'll realise what I've done. I have to get the full vial into me. *Keep going, Tilly. Save yourself, Tilly.*

A siren sounds. Blonde Nurse looks out towards the horizon. She makes a huffing sound and quickly swims away. I can breathe again.

Rational Tilly. Quick. I need to be quick. I withdraw the needle and feel my way to place the plastic safety cap over it. I now have one spare vial of steroid in a little glass ampule. I look around my boat. No more fuel to keep me alive. Rational Tilly. I might need this later. If Blonde Nurse is going to change my sheets and clothes, where can I hide it? I clasp the spare syringe and gently place it down the back of my knickers. They're wet. She might take them off me as well. I nestle the syringe further between my bum cheeks, clenching the muscles tightly together, to hold it in place. What about the glass vial? There's only one place I can think of where it will remain hidden even on the roughest of oceans. My eyes survey the bay. I have no other choice. I slide the tiny glass ampule of lifesaving steroid inside my vagina.

A voice echoes across the ocean.

'What do you think will happen to her?'

Mum. Mum is that you? I call and call. My cries shatter through me and yet, there is no sound. Invisible echoes of fear no one can see or hear.

'She'll probably be sectioned,' Blonde Nurse responds.

Last night, I crossed the liminal boundary into Ward 6, a crack so deep that even the strongest of dandelions would struggle to survive.

This morning, my hospital wristband still reads 'Tilly Rose' but it belongs to a different girl. My vibrant yellow petals have faded into ghostly white strands, so fragile they threaten to be swept away in a single breath. I am bound to this earth only by a wilting stalk, irrepressibly shaking in fear, holding on solely by some primal instinct to stay alive.

I cower in the chair next to my bed, shielding my arms across my face. I am trembling, vulnerable and exposed, a piece of debris swaying in the aftermath of the most violent storm.

'Oh, little one.' Mum stands next to a doctor. They approach me. I recoil, frightened of everyone, frightened of everything.

'Dr Raj would like to say something to you, Tilly,' Mum says.

'I don't know what you remember of last night . . .' he begins.

I remember it all.

'I hear it was very scary, Tilly. I was just telling your mum that, in error, when you moved wards, the glucose and the steroid drips weren't written up. Their sudden removal led to what we call a "hypoxic" episode. This meant your brain wasn't getting enough oxygen. You were right, Tilly. You knew you needed those drips and they should never have been taken away. I really am so sorry.'

'There was a very physical reason for what happened last night,' Mum says. 'You must be terrified, Tilly.'

I don't speak. I can't speak.

'Dr Raj came to assure me that it won't ever happen again but I thought it was really important that *you* heard it from him.'

He nods.

'We've given you an extra bolus of steroid and the drips are now being delivered through your cannula. See here.' He points to a piece of paper. 'Both of the drips are written up. I've repeated them in multiple pages of your notes. So, anytime you feel you need them, Tilly, they're available. Is that OK?'

Nothing is OK and I'm not sure anything will ever be OK again.

PATIENT SURVIVAL TIPS

- Realise that even the pinkest flamingos sometimes need a break.
- Write it down! Keep an up-to-date log of your care plan.
- Physical illnesses can manifest as mental-health problems. Be sure to ask, 'Have you eliminated an organic cause?'
- We are all people before we are patients. Try to find someone who can stand up for the person behind the patient label.
- Lives can be rebuilt, even after the most violent storms.

Part 3
CHAOS

20

TRAPPED

knew I had to save myself. Part of me also knew my mind wasn't working properly. For most of last night, I was trapped in a hellish kaleidoscope of hallucinations, delusions and paranoia, occasionally interrupted by moments of lucidity. Of course, my team never abandoned me. I found out later that Dad, Finn and Auntie were told they had to leave but Mum was allowed to stay on a chair in the corridor outside my bay. She told me that for much of the night, I didn't even know who she was. I banished her from the bed. She forgot to take her handbag; a turn of fate that ultimately saved me. One thing I was not confused about was hearing that word, 'sectioned'. It sliced through me, leaving a jagged wound in its wake.

'Will the hospital be offering Tilly any mental-health support for the mistake last night?' Mum asks today.

Hospitals are, after all, where wounds are stitched up.

'I could offer a referral to her GP for an outpatient follow-up,' the doctor says.

'But she's an inpatient now,' Mum responds.

The doctor awkwardly looks down, unable to hold eye contact.

'I'm afraid our inpatient resources only cover patients who have attempted to commit suicide . . .'

We are constantly told, 'Look after your mental health . . .' 'Ask for help . . .' 'You are not alone . . .' and yet here I am, an inpatient, in a hospital, asking and being told my wound isn't deep enough.

I tell myself I have reached the pit of the well. I can fall no further. Then I do.

Survival mode leaves no time to process the past or look towards the future. I remain stuck in an eternal torturous present on AMU, where patients are usually diagnosed and then sent to the ward specialising in their discipline. The doors of my bay open and close like the turnstiles at an underground station, a continuous loop of people passing through en route to their longer-term, more permanent destinations on the specialist wards. Chest infection = respiratory, heart murmur = cardiology, kidney stones = urology. I have now been stuck here in no-man's land for 31 days. Four porphyria samples have been swallowed up in the abyss of a broken system. We are awaiting test result number 5. Still, no one has diagnosed me. I am stranded on the platform, waiting for a train that never comes.

I may no longer be imprisoned by my mind but I am still a prisoner. I am 'The Girl in the Blue Box', confined by a blue hospital curtain. Any glimpse of natural light is blocked by a faulty window blind. I see the outside world only through bars. My bay is packed so tightly, the next cubicle's chair encroaches on my bed. In the thin gap against the wall, Mum and Auntie push two hard wooden chairs together. Their attempt to construct a makeshift bed is futile; sirens sound, machines bleep, monitors ring out, harrowing screams reverberate through the corridors. One night, at 3am, a fellow patient climbs in my bed. Sleep doesn't belong here.

I think of a little sparrow I once saw trapped on the platform of the underground station. It struck me how incongruent the delicate creature was with its surrounding. Birds are made for skies.

I am now this little sparrow. My nest is a bed of stale sheets, sitting upon on a dirty, blood-stained floor. A television hangs above my head, layered with such a thick film of dust I can etch my name onto the screen. It has a dual use as a makeshift drip stand: there are too few to go around, so my nurse has creatively tied a blue plastic glove around my bottle of IV to suspend it from the TV monitor. The area around my bed hasn't been cleaned since I was moved here, over a month ago.

Lately, my attacks have targeted my tummy, suffocating it in a grip so strong it pins me to the bed. I spend days on end paralysed around my core. Each time an attack ends, my bladder fills as though from nowhere. We ring and ring my call-bell but the ward is a chorus of bells. There aren't enough staff to respond, leaving Mum and Auntie on a constant cleanup cycle. They both have to physically haul me up from my waist and slide bedpans underneath me. They always step outside the blue box to save me that last ounce of dignity, in a world where there is none at all.

The unnatural volumes of urine my body is secreting means the bedpans frequently overflow and the liquid penetrates through the cardboard bases. Even with two people who love me devoted to this task night and day, my bed is surrounded by an undignified moat of leaking cardboard bowls and paper towels. We are living in a communal toilet. The bins are constantly overflowing. There is nowhere to dispose of them and no one to take them away. In the bathroom, next to the sink, other patients' bedpans stack up, filled with urine and faeces. I'm a sparrow with two companions in my nest but what about the sparrows trapped here all alone?

'Can I please go to the toilet?' the lady diagonally across from me asks.

'Go in your nappy,' a nurse shouts back.

'But I can walk to the toilet. I just need an arm or a frame to get there.'

'We're too busy, just go in your nappy.'

This morning, Mum asks the nurse if someone can log that I'm producing extreme amounts of urine.

'This can't be normal.' She points to the moat around my bed. 'We keep asking if someone can monitor it.'

'You're best to ask one of the regular nurses. I'm just agency,' she shrugs.

Agency nurses are called in last minute to deal with the overwhelming staff shortages across the hospital. AMU seems to be constantly short-staffed, which means agency nurses on every shift. It also means new nurses. They have no sense of who I was when I arrived here or who I am now. I am just 'Bed 3'.

'Do you have a towel Tilly could use please?' Auntie asks.

She's trying to give me a bed bath, with a wet flannel and some soap she's brought from home.

The nurse returns a few minutes later. She hands over a pillowcase.

'Can only find this, I'm afraid.'

'Thank you so much,' I say. I am in a hospital, grateful that I have been given a pillowcase to dry myself with.

'All clean again.' Auntie smiles a sad smile. She hands me her little pocket mirror. The reflection is a girl I struggle to recognise. Her skinny face and body have ballooned. None of her clothes fit around her anymore. She is like a toxic tank, filling and filling with water. Her blonde hair has turned brown. It sticks to her head, scraped back in a scraggly knot. Her sallow eyes peep out under a tapestry of anaesthetic patches. Her skin is tattooed with bruises; some are purple and round, others spray painted in dark blue and reds. The most arresting are the faded yellows, ageing over time. One cannula hangs from her right arm, another from her left hand and a third from her foot. They are haphazardly stuck down with masking tape. Their rough edges peel away exposing grimy, grey corners. Only one cannula still works but the old ones remain. Her wristband fell off weeks ago. It was never replaced. She is no longer Tilly Rose.

Day and night, I watch people come and go, but there is one passenger who remains stuck on the platform with me. Leena, the patient in the next bed, has been here since that first night I arrived on AMU. She has become my constant in an everchanging scene.

'This was me, just two days before I was admitted here.' She stretches her arm across the thin aisle between our two beds to show me a photograph. In it, she is out for lunch with two friends to celebrate her 60th birthday, sitting outside in a courtyard, bathed in summer sun. Her thick, dark hair frames her beaming face. She looks so healthy, so alive. I struggle to reconcile this image with the lady I see lying beside me. Her once sparkling eyes are now sunken, her vibrant skin now papery and dry, her rich, glossy hair now matted and grey. Occasionally, her warm smile peeps through, giving me a fleeting glimpse of the lady in the photograph but it's becoming rarer with each day that passes.

With just a thin curtain between us, we hear each other's struggles play out in real time.

'We were told the cancer required *urgent* medical treatment *six weeks ago*,' I hear Leena's daughter, Safa, say. 'But six weeks on, she still hasn't started *any* treatment.'

'I think it's already been explained to you. We know she has both kidney and liver cancer but the problem is, we still don't know which is the *primary* cancer,' the doctor responds. 'That determines which team she gets put under. If the kidney is the primary, it will be nephrology and if the liver is the primary, it will be hepatology.'

This discussion has been going on for weeks. Each day, I will Safa to keep going, to keep standing up for her mum. Leena is now too unwell to fight for her own life. Her daughter is her only hope.

'I can see how day one it might have been important to work out the primary cancer, but six weeks on Mum's really deteriorating. Surely it no longer makes sense to keep waiting. Can one team please just take ownership and start the chemo?'

'I'll chase the biopsy result again today and discuss it with the teams again,' the doctor says.

'We're told this every day but nothing changes. If there's a problem with the sample, please let's take another one. We need to move this forward.'

'I do understand your frustration,' the doctor says.

'Mum's now had two infections, developed ascites and is rapidly losing weight. She'll be too weak for the chemo if we wait much longer.' I can hear Safa's internal silent screams. I feel like screaming with her. Leena has fallen victim to a medical system that relies on putting people in boxes. While she awaits the doctors' verdict, she's withering away in the confines of her own blue box.

'I'll make sure someone updates you later,' the doctor says.

Safa steps out of Leena's cubicle and turns to Mum.

'I'm not doing enough for her. We're going around in circles.' A tear rolls down her cheek. She wipes it away.

'That's not true, Safa.' Mum squeezes her hand and looks over at Leena. 'You have a wonderful daughter, don't you, Leena?'

Leena manages a brief smile and slight nod. Safa has taken two months off work so she can constantly be by her mum's side.

'If they fire me, they fire me. If we end up having to go privately and sell the house to pay for her care, we'll sell the house. All that matters is Mum,' she said to us, the first time we met.

She now flits between roles as a full-time carer, showering Leena with unwavering love, and a part-time medical researcher, poised with her laptop, ready to log every conversation with every doctor. She questions everything and takes nothing as fact; but Leena, like me, is hovering in no-man's land, slipping through a system that insists on binary categories.

'Who gives a fuck which came first?' Safa mutters. 'Why can't they just get on and treat her?'

In the weeks spent living alongside Leena and her family, we've developed a unique bond. With my attacks spiralling and not enough staff to keep up with the level of care I'm requiring, Mum and Auntie have been allowed to stay. Some nights they alternate, but recently, things have become so bad, it has taken both of them. I sometimes go for stretches of 72 hours with no sleep at all. If my body ever calms for just a few minutes, Mum curls up at the end of my bed and Auntie balances on the makeshift chairs. They have become Safa's eyes and ears on the ward at night.

'It's my only comfort, knowing you're here to look out for Mum at night. I hate the thought of her being alone.'

'We'll always look out for her, Safa. We're up all night with Tilly and we always check on Leena.'

'You would phone me, wouldn't you, if you were concerned?'

'I promise,' Mum nods.

This afternoon, Safa's sister, Calla, and brother, Fadi, enter the ward, carrying boxes full of fresh salads, meats and bottles of cold pressed juices.

'We've made you a Syrian feast, Mum,' Fadi says.

'Can I tempt you to try some balouza, Tilly?' He walks over to my bedside, holding a box of colourful desserts in delicate little pots.

This gesture makes my day.

Then he turns to Safa and hands her a steaming paper cup.

'A tea for you.'

Calla wraps her arms around her sister, then stands back and wipes a tear from her cheek. She gives her a steely nod, as if to say, 'Keep going; stay strong for Mum.' Like us, they are a team. When one team member crumbles, the others are there to pick them up.

Mondays on AMU have become the day of the week that fills me with dread. Each Monday a different consultant enters the ward. It's a total lottery in terms of who they are and where their specialism lies. They do their one-week stint and then move on. Some consultants appear on a Monday morning, never to be seen again. Juniors are regularly abandoned to the chaos of the ward, with no one to guide them.

On other wards, patients benefit from the continuity of care from specialist teams who understand their condition and see them regularly, but everything about AMU – including the patients – is supposed to be temporary. Now, on day 45 of my stay, I am starting to feel like an unwelcome guest at a party I never chose to attend.

This Monday's consultant, Dr Muncher, stands at the end of my bed.

'It's been a busy one so far today. One dead, one dying and now you.'

It seems Dr Muncher missed the Bedside Manner seminar at med school.

'I've just read through your case notes,' he says.

Every Monday, the new consultant on AMU is faced with my ever-growing case history. Given that Muncher's already been extremely busy this morning dealing with the 'dead' and 'dying', I wonder when he's found the time to fit in all this reading.

'How long have you been here?' he asks.

Ah – skim-reading, then.

'Forty-five days . . .'

'And I understand there's a perceived inability to walk, perceived abdominal swelling, perceived head pain . . .'

I stare up at him in disbelief.

'Perceived?'

He looks back at me quizzically.

'Perceived,' I repeat. 'You just used the word "perceived" three times when describing my symptoms.'

'Did I?'

The junior next to him looks down, unable to hold my gaze.

'Yes, you did,' I say. 'Can you please explain why?'

'Well, all the tests are normal.'

My silent scream threatens to soar to the surface after weeks, months, *years* of being trodden down. I feel I am about to break and yet I know that doing so will only strengthen the assumptions Muncher has already made about me. So, instead, I take a breath and, in a calm, even voice, I do the only thing I can do: I question the logic.

'I'm saying my head is agony and you can see there are two swellings on it. I'm saying my abdomen is locking and you can see I look pregnant. I'm saying my muscles are being attacked and you can visibly see them vibrating. I'm saying my feet are burning and you can see pustules erupting through the skin. How can these symptoms be "perceived" when they are so overtly visible?'

He carries on as if I've said nothing at all.

'Have you been getting up and about?'

I shake my head.

'Well, what's stopping you?'

Did Muncher not hear a single word of what I just said? I try again.

'The attacks, the episodes of paralysis, the convulsions, the pain . . .'

'Well, you're not having them now,' he interrupts. 'Do you want to be in hospital, Tilly?'

I look around the blue box.

'Why would *anyone* want to live *here*?'

'I can see you're deconditioned. We need to get you on the move.'

'I really do want to be out of this bed but moving always brings on an attack . . .'

'Let's see, shall we?'

Auntie returns holding a coffee.

'Good timing: we're just off on a walk,' Muncher grins. 'Will you be joining us?'

I talk to Auntie through my eyes. Like me, she knows that this is a terrible idea; but, like me, she also knows I have to be seen to be 'trying'. She leans over to support my crumpled, quivering body from the bed. Each step forward is like wading through a swamp. My feet are sucked down by the thick, squelching mud. I strain through the marshy reeds. The further I push on, the more the stagnant water rises.

'Now for the stairs.' Muncher pushes the double doors open to reveal a decaying staircase below.

He leads me into the swamp. Then, five steps down, he suddenly has to dash.

'Auntie can take over now.'

Muncher doesn't wait to see my shrivelled, eroding body wash up on his shore. He doesn't witness the ravaging attack that ensues within minutes of returning to my bed. He doesn't hear me crying out. The swamp lingers but Muncher has gone.

Monday morning comes around again. Leena and I watch on longingly as the lady in the bed opposite is discharged. A pharmacist arrives to dispense her meds and check her care plan.

'We see you live alone, Hettie.'

'No, I don't.' Hettie shakes her head firmly.

'According to your notes, you've lived by yourself for a few years now . . .'

'I told you: I don't live on my own.'

'We're only checking so we can be sure you'll manage OK back at home. Otherwise, we may need to arrange some extra help for a little while.'

'I've lived with Daniel since 1986.'

'Oh, right, there's nothing in our records about a Daniel.'

It turns out Daniel doesn't feature in the records because Daniel is, in fact, a tortoise.

Leena turns her head to face me. We catch eyes and smile, grasping onto a rare flicker of light relief, a snapshot of another world.

The moment is snatched away by the sound of footsteps, followed by a tap on my hospital curtain. When this Monday's consultant appears, I have no expectations. I have learned that if I have no expectations, I can't be let down. There's only so much one heart can take.

'Hello, Tilly, I'm Dr Day,' he smiles. 'But call me Jack.'

'Are you Tilly's family?' he turns to Mum and Auntie, who are squished up against the wall, forever attempting to appear invisible, fearful that at any moment they could be made to leave.

He introduces himself to them, then turns back to me.

'So, I've read through your notes.'

Here we go again . . .

'There are a lot. Sorry I'm a bit later getting to you today. It's taken me a while to piece them all together.'

He jumps into a rapid stream-of-consciousness, giving voice to every thought, every connection and every theory that pops into his brain. It turns out he really has read my notes, all 51 days' worth. He's also memorised them in intricate detail. Jack has questions, lots of them.

'You're no doubt an expert on these attacks, Tilly – can you describe them to me?'

I gabble away, ready to be interrupted, to be cut short. It doesn't happen. Jack listens when I speak. Then, he turns to Mum and Auntie to include them in the conversation.

'I'm sure you've seen far more of Tilly over the last few weeks than any of the doctors. Family often notice things the doctors may not have picked up on. I want to know any details you may think are relevant.'

I catch eyes with Mum and give her a 'What's going on?' look. This isn't what we're used to. Mum hands him a list of my ever-growing symptoms. He asks if he can make a copy. Mum then invites him to attend the movie premiere of my 'live attack'. So far, on this ward, no one has been interested in watching her film clip. She looks surprised when Jack takes a seat, fully absorbed from start to finish. He even takes notes.

'This is really useful evidence, thank you.'

Evidence. I like that word. I need a detective to solve my case. At the same time, I'm scared to trust him. My trust has been broken too many times before.

'I keep craving apple juice,' I say, bracing myself to be dismissed.

'How peculiar.' He pauses for a moment. 'Any particular variety? Clear or cloudy?'

Is he humouring me? I don't think so. His face remains sincere.

'Cloudy. Pink Lady, actually.'

'It could be the smallest detail that proves the most relevant,' he says, noting it down. He clicks onto the computer, flashing up a set of results. 'Now, what's most significant about this admission so far is your lactate levels.'

I glance up, unsure what he's referring to.

'Your lactate recently reached 11. I'm not sure how you are still alive.'

His words beat through me like a solid punch winding my stomach. Why has no one mentioned these results? Mum slides onto the mattress beside me and squeezes my shoulder. A rush of fear pulses through me. I stop it in its tracks. Jack is only confirming what I've consistently been saying: each attack *feels* like a death sentence. This is validation. Now someone else is confirming what I've known all along. Each attack *is* a death sentence.

'And yet here you are,' he adds.

270

I manage a slight smile. I'm still here. That's something.

'Your body is in some way saving itself, Tilly. The question is: how?'

After so long in here, I've started to dream about getting a positive result. It's not that I *want* to be ill. It's that I know I *am* ill and 'normal' test results give us nothing to work with. At last, I have results to prove how ill I really am. It shouldn't have to be this way and yet, I know that in medicine *everything* rests on test results.

'You must be feeling very unwell,' Jack says.

He gives me the acknowledgement I've been yearning for.

'Have these lactate results been consistently high, then?' Mum asks.

Whenever we ask for a copy of my results, we're told to formally apply online through the 'patient portal'. The first obstacle is that this requires a passport (naturally top of most patients' packing list) and the second is that the results can then take up to 30 days to come through. What use is the knowledge that you have life-threatening lactate levels after you've been discharged or, worse still, once you're already dead?

'Yes, levels of 8, 9, 10, 11.'

I feel a strange mixture of fear and validation.

'With these lactate levels, I would have expected you to have gone into full-blown lactic acidosis, where dangerous levels of acid build up in the blood. I've worked out that in order for you to still be alive, your body must be compensating by taking a strange pathway to prevent this from happening.'

Mum explains how everyone seems to think I have porphyria but we still don't have a result.

'It's definitely an option, but sometimes we can become too narrow with our focus. What happens is, every medic who reads your notes sees the word "porphyria" and then their thinking all plays into this bias. It's important we keep our minds open to other things.'

He makes a good point. He makes lots of good points.

Mum flips over another page in her notebook and tentatively begins her usual effort to make us heard.

'Obviously I'm not a doctor, but I am a desperate mum. I've been researching and have a few ideas that maybe I could put to you . . .'

He gestures for her to share them. She hands over a piece of paper with a bullet-point list of possible diagnoses and test suggestions, with a sentence next to each point explaining why she thinks it fits. He runs his finger down the page.

'Yes, Fanconi is a possibility . . . No, that next one doesn't explain the lactate . . . Yes, cytochrome P450 and steroid genesis could be relevant . . .'

I'm mystified by the scene taking place. He doesn't disregard Mum as 'the patient's mother'; he sees she's sharing logical, well-researched, relevant information that is going to help solve this. Jack treats her and all of us as part of his team.

I've never met a medic like him. In one way, he's like a human computer but he also has a heart. He finishes by recapping not only the tests he plans to arrange but also how it's essential that, in the meantime, they ease my symptoms to make me feel a little better.

'I see you still haven't been referred to the pain team after almost two months.' He holds his hand to his brow, shaking his head.

Every second of every day, the pain is eroding more of me away. I know that even if someone could just take the edge off it, I would have more strength to fight another day. When Jack says he'll be asking them to visit, I want to cry. A *whole team* devoted to pain. Bring it on.

'You haven't had any physio either?'

I shake my head. His expression, once again, says, 'This is ludicrous,' but also, 'I'm not surprised.' We share a knowing look.

'Your body is too unwell to cope with anything strenuous at present.' I think of Muncher, only last week, dragging me to the stairs. 'But maybe the physio could help you with a few bed exercises, so you still have some muscle at the end of this.'

The end of this. He thinks there will be an *end* of this.

'Yes, please. Anything, anything at all you can offer.'

'Thank you, thank you so much,' we all repeat over and over.

After he leaves, I look towards Mum and Auntie, disbelief painted across our faces. He's like no doctor I have ever come across. I don't want to trust him and yet, everything about him instils trust.

'He's, he's . . .' I begin, unable to find the words.

'A maverick,' Auntie replies.

PATIENT SURVIVAL TIPS

- When healthcare professionals dismiss or minimise your informed concerns about your health, it can make you doubt your own reality – this is known as medical gaslighting, and it's never OK.
- If you are presented with something illogical, always question the logic.
- Find your voice.
- Value anyone who is trying to help.
- Give the bud of hope a chance.

21

MAVERICK

Sometimes, when all hope is lost, someone comes along who restores our faith in humanity. Over the next week, Maverick does all the things he says he's going to do: he reviews my whole medical history, he contacts doctors whose care I've been under previously, he stays late at night to research my case, he organises new tests, he arranges for the pain team and physio to visit, he contacts specialist units at other hospitals and shares ideas of further investigations. Maverick sees a zebra in front of him and takes the time to analyse every stripe.

'And what do *you* think this could be?' Mum asks.

The amount of time, thought and research Maverick has invested in my case, means his opinion is now the one that matters.

'Well, piecing it all together, the only two things I think fit are either porphyria, which we are still awaiting a result on, or one of the other ideas I have is heavy metal poisoning,' he says.

'*Heavy metal poisoning?*' I look up at him. 'How could I have that?'

'I don't know exactly, but we have to look at all the possibilities.'

Each time Maverick pops his head into my cubicle, the space is filled with a new kind of energy, because every time he enters, he offers something new.

'Why are you helping Tilly?' Mum asks.

Maverick waves his hand, as if to say, 'It's nothing.'

'As a mother, it is everything,' Mum responds.

For weeks, we have been trapped under the weight of a thick, smoggy sky, so polluted that it was concealing even the brightest stars. Just one glimmer of light across this dark, futile landscape has reinvigorated not just me but my whole team to keep believing.

I think of Mum's words: 'It only takes one person. Only one person needs to care, Tilly.'

'We're so grateful for the time you're spending thinking about Tilly's case. We realise it's very complicated,' Auntie says.

'It would be a lot easier if she were on my ward,' Maverick responds.

'Could I move?' A flicker of hope ignites inside me. This could change everything.

'Sadly, the system won't allow it. I'm a consultant on the respiratory ward and you haven't been diagnosed with a respiratory condition.'

'I did have TB . . .'

'But you don't have it now. This is something else.' He shakes his head, despondently. 'There are still lots of avenues for us to pursue, though, Tilly, so I better get to work.'

I look up at this man and see the compassion in his eyes. Kindness alone won't make me better; but *thinking* and kindness, now that is a winning combination.

'You're a different sort of doctor,' I say to Maverick, as he leaves.

He smiles and says, 'I try.'

'The porphyria test has come back negative,' Dr Richardson, this Monday's consultant, tells me.

It felt like everything rested on this result.

'Can we trust it?' I ask.

'Yes. You've had eight tests and they've all come back negative.'

'But seven were compromised,' I say.

'We can't do any more,' he responds.

'On the basis that the medics have told us Tilly has all the symptoms of porphyria, could she try the treatment, which I understand is called "heme", anyway?' Mum asks.

'We have to draw a line under it,' Dr Richardson says.

'But what if you gave it to her and she got better?' Mum poses.

'Even if she was dying in ICU, the system wouldn't allow us to give her the heme treatment without a positive porphyria result.'

His words echo through me, submerging me further into the depths of fear and despair.

'We're now scraping the barrel for tests,' he says.

Auntie leans over and squeezes my hand.

'Last week's consultant had lots of suggestions for new test ideas,' Auntie says. 'Could someone maybe speak to him?'

'He's back on his own ward with his own patients now,' Dr Richardson informs us. Maverick wanted me to be on his ward with him but the system wouldn't allow it. With that, all of his promising ideas and plans are lost to the no-man's land of AMU.

'At some point we have to decide enough is enough,' Dr Richardson says.

On day one, doctors stood patiently at my bedside, wanting to know every detail, watching on with tears in their eyes. Over two months on, I still have no diagnosis. It's starting to feel like I'm in some way to blame.

'You can't just carry on living here forever,' Dr Richardson adds.

I take in the stifling ward that I dream of escaping, every second of every day. This isn't living, it's surviving.

When Dr Richardson leaves, Auntie turns to me, a melancholy look in her eyes.

'I'm so sorry, Tilly. You really are a zebra in a horse hospital.'

A few hours later, a man with grey hair, a checked shirt and navy chinos pops his head around my curtain. For a second, I dare to hope that a fresh pair of eyes has been sent to review my case.

'Hello.' He gives me a little nod.

'Hello,' I reply.

'I hear you've been feeling disassociated,' the man says.

I look up at him, confused. What's he talking about?

'Sorry, I'm not sure I caught who you are?' Auntie says.

He could have quite literally walked in here off the street.

'I'm a psychiatrist.'

Still no name.

He turns to me.

'Do you think you're made of wood?'

I stare up at him, my head tilted to the side, my face scrunched in total, absolute bewilderment.

'Sorry? *Wood*, as in wood from trees?'

He nods, as if this is the most natural question in the world. I must have misunderstood.

'Erm no, I don't think I'm made of wood.'

He nods.

'Plastic?'

The next logical step. I look up at him again, perplexed. He waits.

'Erm, no, I don't think I'm made of plastic either.'

He writes something down.

'I understand your family and partner have been visiting. Do you think they are real?'

'Yes,' I respond, without missing a beat. I look towards Auntie squashed in the chair beside me. 'They are my team.'

Auntie gives me a sad smile, her eyes willing me to keep going.

'Dr Richardson said you've been feeling a bit disassociated,' Dr No-Name informs me.

'No, I never said that. I said I had a strange electric feeling in my head . . .'

'Right, well, I don't think you are disassociated but I will have to return tomorrow to conduct a full psychiatric report. Is that OK?'

I stare up at him, unable to gather my thoughts. After my terrifying night of psychosis, no psychological assessment or support could be offered – but now that weeks on no *physical* diagnosis has been made and I'm continuing to take up a bed,

Dr No-Name has been sent for multiple visits. The predictability is what's most frightening of all.

Three days later, the psychiatry report concludes that there is no psychological cause of my symptoms. It concludes what I have known all along. There is a physical cause. It just hasn't been found yet.

'I can't keep doing it,' I say when today's attack finally begins to calm, and yet some part of me knows I will keep doing it. I will do it as many times as it needs to be done.

It's a weird contradiction: during my most acute attacks, I am in such agony I want it all to be over and yet, in those same moments, my biggest fear is actually dying. Instinctively, I jump into survival mode and fight with everything I have to stay alive.

It is in the stretches of time in between the attacks, when the acuteness dampens down a little and I am trapped in a chronic state of torture, that I question how I will continue. I am a hot potato, teetering on the edge of boiling point night and day. Nothing touches the heat. Nothing touches the pain. My team buy me a fan. They get creative; Dad and Finn wrap ice cubes in blue plastic gloves and place them behind my neck. They resort to buying large bags of ice from the supermarket next to the hospital. I lie on top of them, letting them soak through my searing flank and penetrate my clothes. It is in this state that living becomes scary.

'I can't live like this; I can't do it,' I say.

'You won't have to, Tilly, because it won't be like this forever,' Finn says.

I look up at this boy I was so scared to let in on day one, now leaning over me to remove a bedpan full of my urine like it's the most normal thing in the world.

'Finn, this is so beyond normal. No one would judge you for walking away.' This is hardly what you picture when conjuring up a scene of 'young love'. So far, Mum and Auntie have always been here for these undignified outbursts but I've now been caught short while they've headed out to the main entrance to grab a gulp of fresh air.

'I'm exactly where I need to be,' Finn responds.

'You can't *want* to be here; you can't love this,' I say.

'Of course I don't love this.' He looks around the chaotic ward.

'Exactly, so go – you have a choice, Finn.'

'I don't,' he says.

'You do.'

'I don't, because I love you.'

I hold his gaze as his words sink in. Never before have I felt so much like the spider in the web. I panic that Finn is now permanently entangled in my silk threads, trapped by my side in this living hell, struggling to find a way out.

'But why?' I wave my hand down the body of this girl I no longer recognise.

'Well, that's simple, Tilly. You're easy to love.'

He stands up, taking away the leaking bedpan in a handful of tissues. Day one, this scene was unimaginable – I didn't even want to admit to Finn that I was ill – but over the years, we've grown into this warped reality together. We've done the good times but also the bad, the sickness and the health, and we're still here. Deep down,

I know we're bound not by a web of guilt but by an unbreakable bond of love.

Suddenly, a harrowing scream erupts down the corridor. It belongs to a male patient who howls night and day. I now have a sense of what it is to be trapped in your own mind; to be trapped there permanently must be a dark and lonely place. I *feel* his cries.

'Can we go somewhere else?' I whisper to Finn when he returns to my cubicle.

The tormented wails echo through my bay.

'Where do you want to go, Tilly?'

'Home,' I whisper.

He nods, then leans forward to hold my hands in his.

'OK, it's Sunday morning. The sun is streaming through the windows of our flat. A pile of newspapers and magazines lie on the window seat. We sip on frothy coffees, looking out at the blue sky. The radio is playing happy weekend tunes in the background . . .'

For a few blissful moments, I savour the magic of ordinary life, before being thrown back into the chaos of the ward.

'Brian, stand back from the door,' Nurse Indira shouts from the corridor.

Our bay is now under attack. A male patient, in nothing but a gown, has made his way down the corridor and is attempting to bash down our door with his walking stick. Finn hovers between mine and Leena's bed, our only protection as we lie flat on our backs, helpless to escape.

Through the window, I take in all 6ft 4in of Brian and all 5ft 3in of Indira. In one swift move, Brian flings his arms across Indira's head, swiping her glasses off her face. She dives to the floor at the precise moment backup arrives.

Minutes later, Indira walks into our bay, holding her broken glasses.

'That's a whole shift for nothing,' she says.

'Can you not claim it back?' Finn asks.

'There's so much paperwork it's not worth it.' She shrugs despondently.

Ordinary life doesn't exist in here for patients, or for staff.

PATIENT SURVIVAL TIPS

- 'Who are you?' is a perfectly legitimate question to ask anyone who appears at the end of your bed.
- Practical hacks can be game-changing for coping with symptoms.
- If you can't escape your surroundings, let your mind take you elsewhere.
- We are bound by love, not by guilt.
- You are still here, reading this now. Your own chapters are still being written.

22

HOLD ON

This afternoon, Mum is sitting beside me when there is a light tap on my curtain.

'Hello, my name is Ava.' I glance up to see a lady with a short bob and warm smile. 'I'm a volunteer from the hospital chaplaincy. I was wondering if you might like to chat?'

It's a lovely idea but not very me. It feels a bit awkward to turn her away, though.

'Of course,' I murmur.

Ava begins to explain how the hospital chaplaincy service offers a listening ear to any patient who would like to talk, whatever their beliefs. I definitely wouldn't like to talk but listening to Ava provides a momentary distraction, so I ask her a few questions. I'm intrigued when she tells me she's a humanist.

'It's mostly about being kind on this earth,' she says to me.

I realise Ava isn't on a mission to convert me; she isn't on a mission to do anything, other than to be kind. The more she talks, the more I like her. When she asks if I'd be happy for her to pop in again, I'm surprised to find myself saying yes – and not because I feel I should but because I'd actually like to see her again.

'How about I leave you to it?' Mum suggests the third time Ava pops by. The thought of being alone with someone actively trying to make me talk, without Mum as a buffer, would usually send me into panic mode, but that's just the thing: Ava doesn't try. She just chats to me like we're friends. I start to open up, not because I'm being told I should but because I want to.

Mum heads off and Ava takes a seat beside me.

'How are you today, Tilly?'

'OK,' I say.

She pauses for a second.

'How are you really?'

'Not good.' Sometimes you need someone to ask the next question, to give you permission to say what's really going on inside. 'Ever since that terrifying night of hypoxia, I've lost trust in everything about this place,' I say. 'And now, a month on, I'm still imprisoned in the same blue box, where it all took place. It's tormenting me.'

'It must feel like torture, Tilly,' Ava says.

I nod.

'Can you not ask to be moved?'

'I have, lots of times.'

I pause. I'm stuck on the bed, gripping my yellow cushion to my locked tummy. There isn't a single second of the day where I am not aware of the agonising pain. My only respite is sleep but even that is rare. I still spend stretches of up to 72 hours awake. This illness is unrelenting.

'I don't think I can keep doing it,' I say to Ava.

'I believe you can do it, Tilly.'

The girl who arrived here believed that too, but so much has happened since then.

I take in Ava's soft, gentle expression. I realise I trust her. I can talk to her in a way that is usually solely reserved for my team. Over the course of this admission, Mum, Dad, Finn and Auntie have stayed so strong for me; but I know inside they are crumbling. We are all crumbling. Each of us has had to put up a wall, in order to survive. There is still one fear that remains unspoken even to them, a fear I have sometimes cried out during an attack but never explicitly discussed.

I glance towards Ava. It somehow feels less daunting to share it with someone outside of our little unit.

'I'm frightened it's going to kill me,' I whisper.

The words hang in the air between us. I look down, unable to meet her eyes.

Ava leans towards me.

'That must be terrifying, Tilly.'

I give a slight nod, swallowing back my tears.

'You are incredibly brave. I know you don't have a choice.'

'I don't want to be brave anymore,' I say.

'You shouldn't have to be, but you can't give up now.'

'I'm scared one of the attacks is going to kill me before they find the cause.' My voice quivers. With each familiar wave of sweat that envelops my body, signalling the beginning of an attack, I never know whether it will be the one that gets me.

'How many of these attacks have you had now Tilly?' Ava asks after a pause.

'Too many to count.'

'And you're still here.' She gestures over to me.

I look down at my trembling muscles, my raw, inflamed skin and my withering limbs.

'I don't know how. My body doesn't work.'

'Tilly, you've survived all of this. Your body has saved you again and again. I think you have a very strong body.'

I tilt my head to the side, staring out through the slit of light in the faulty window blind. Internally, I've been berating my body for weeks, asking why, whatever I do, it still won't work; wishing it could just fit the textbook and stop presenting in ways that no one understands. I've felt let down by my body. I've blamed it for making me suffer.

'You are *not* your illness, Tilly.'

I mull on Ava's words. She allows me to see that my body and this illness are entirely separate. I imagine the illness racing through my blood, armed with weapons and explosions. I am just the vessel it has, unfortunately, decided to land in. It's succeeding in its mission to make me really frightened. It's succeeding in its mission to make me feel I am going to die.

Ava pauses for a moment, then turns to the photo frame on my windowsill.

'Tell me about this girl.'

It's a photo of me, beaming in a pink dress at a family party with my best friend Florrie. Our mums went to school together and I've known Florrie since the day I was born. Ava asks me details about the day – where the party was held, what we ate, what we drank, who was there. For a few blissful minutes, I am not 'The Girl in the Blue Box', lying flat on the hospital bed, bruises littering her skin, cannulas hanging from her arms and pain patches covering her face, I am 'The Girl in the Pink Dress'.

'You have so much love around you, Tilly,' Ava smiles. She gestures to the abundance of cards lining my windowsill. There are so many, we've now taped them in rows up the wall. A rainbow of colour in a bleak landscape.

I tell Ava how my friends have dropped in homemade cakes, meals on wheels, celery juice and last-minute coffees on their way to work. I tell her how Auntie Geraldine has filled our freezer with homemade dinners and how my inbox is always bursting with words of love. None of them stop messaging, even though I'm too ill to reply. The part that means the most is the consistency. They've all continued to rally around, not only during those first few weeks but months on.

'Have you seen any of your friends since being in here?' Ava asks. I shake my head.

'Well, only my friend Nina weeks ago, before she moved to Norway. I don't want anyone to see me like this.'

'Are you allowed to go outside, Tilly?' Ava asks.

'I don't know.' It's not something I've even considered, most of the time I'm too ill to even move from the bed.

'I think it might help to connect with the world beyond the hospital window.' She points to the photo of me in the pink dress. 'It's important to keep this girl alive.'

For months, two parallel lives have stagnated. On each side of the hospital curtain, my neighbour Leena and I have become inextricably connected, stuck together in the perpetual no-man's land of AMU.

Meanwhile, the world beyond our window keeps moving. Last week, my friend Florrie gave birth to a beautiful baby girl, Isla. When she suggests bringing her to meet me at the main entrance of the hospital, it feels incomprehensible. Each day, Isla awakens to an eternal dawn of new beginnings. Whereas death and trauma linger in the very air I breathe.

'She's desperate to meet her Auntie Tilly,' Florrie messages.

For a moment, l allow myself to imagine holding Isla in my arms and no longer being 'Tilly the patient' but being 'Auntie Tilly'. I ponder on this for days, Ava's words reverberating through me: 'keep this girl alive'.

This afternoon, overcome by a surge of courage, I finally agree to make the momentous trip down to the main entrance. I've dreamed of escaping this place for so long but now that I'm faced with the reality, I'm paralysed with fear. There's a familiarity within the hell that I've come to cling onto. I know I can survive here, in this blue box, because I've done it time and time again; but out there, uncertainty prevails.

'Uncertainty also offers possibility,' Mum reminds me.

The girl who arrived here wasn't frightened by what-ifs, but I am a different girl now. I've learned that uncertainty can also conceal threats that appear without warning.

'I can't do it,' I whisper, cowering back in the wheelchair.

Across the curtain, I watch Safa lean over Leena, stroking her mum's cheek with tenderness and love. She looks up and catches my eye.

'You've got this, Tilly.'

Only now do I take in the scene playing out beside me. Safa is sitting with her mum, while Calla and Fadi gather Leena's belongings and pack them into bags.

'Mum's . . . being moved to a side room,' Safa whispers.

Leena's family have been asking for her to be moved for weeks – this is what they've all been yearning for, but now the moment is here there are no smiles. Instead, a thick, suffocating silence hangs around the bed. I take in Leena's weak, exhausted body strewn across the sheets. I look from Safa to Fadi to Calla and then up to Mum. Their eyes are filled with tears. It hits me. Still, no one has identified the *primary* cancer. Still, no department has taken ownership of Leena's case. Still, she hasn't started any treatment.

I'm about to escape the ward to glimpse the outside world. I'm frightened by the prospect of an uncertain future and yet, as I look over at Leena, fading away, I am certain of one thing. When I return to the ward, her bed will be empty. I will never see her again.

My breathing becomes rapid as we approach the doors to the main entrance. I shrink back into the rickety wheelchair, shielding my hands in front of my face. I feel like I've been plonked in a scene, without a script. I don't know how to occupy the world out here.

'I can't let Florrie see me like this.'

I realise I'm not only scared about going outside; I'm also scared of what the outside world will make of me. It feels silly to care about what I look like in the wake of what I've been through and yet, my swollen face and heavy body torment me. In recent weeks, despite barely eating, I have put on over 12kg in fluid. My puffy eyes, my tight skin and ballooning tummy mean I no longer look like *me*. My skin remains tattooed with deep purple bruises and crusty scabs. It tells the story of an endless, painful search for veins. The venomous red snake riddling my feet continues to spiral in angry circles. My muscles have wasted. My limbs are littered with cannulas, smeared with blood. Dirty masking tape peels back at the corners, leaving sticky lines of grey glue. My face is barely visible under the anaesthetic pain patches. More plasters line my calves and flank. My hair is pulled back in a matted knot. The only part of me that remains from my life before is a fleck of orange nail varnish, a relic of my former self.

Mum kneels down beside me and holds my hand.

'What are you worried Florrie's going to think?' she asks.

Before I can answer, I hear a voice calling my name. Standing in the mellow, autumn sun, at the front of the hospital, is Florrie. In her arms is newborn Isla.

Mum wheels me towards them. I came in here in the blaze of the summer heatwave. Now, the leaves have turned burnt orange and are falling from the trees. The crisp air fills my lungs. I look across at the benches at the main entrance awash with other patients, identifiable with gowns and wristbands and lines hanging from their limbs. Over the wall, normal life resumes. Cars drive past, customers bob in and out of coffee shops, people cross the street. I quiver and recoil back into my chair. I don't belong here.

Florrie tilts her head to the side and properly takes me in. A single look will never reveal what I've been through and yet, a single look is enough to touch her heart. A tear rolls down her cheek.

I see myself through Florrie's gaze, not as a patient but as a human being. Someone's friend, someone's daughter, someone's partner, desperately clinging onto life. This isn't what people imagine when they think of 'hope'; but hope isn't gentle – it's visceral and raw. This is what hope really looks like.

'Someone has been desperate to meet you. Would you like to hold her, Auntie Tilly?' Florrie asks.

My lip trembles. I instinctively pull away. Florrie is existing in her happy bubble with her newborn baby. My story will permeate their pages and leave a lasting stain.

'Go on,' Mum whispers softly.

I shake my head. Here are two worlds that shouldn't collide.

'Please give me a cuddle, Auntie Tilly,' Florrie says, turning Isla towards me.

I slowly stretch my head up, my face scrunched in timid fear. I give a slight nod. Florrie leans down and places Isla onto my lap. I gasp, as she wraps her tiny little fingers around mine. My life inside the blue box has stagnated but now in my arms is a bundle of infinite possibility. Baby Isla reminds me that the world beyond my window is constantly evolving and with that comes progress and the possibility of change.

When I return to my bed, Leena and her family are gone. It seems incomprehensible that only two months ago we were complete strangers, leading entirely separate lives. Like me, Leena wouldn't allow anyone but her closest family to gather around her hospital bed. For the last two months, with just a thin curtain between us, we had no choice but to let each other in. We were two shards of glass swept together in a merciless storm. Our chapters played out in tandem as we battled a system intent on trying to fit us into boxes. With no one taking ownership, we both remained stuck in an eternal stasis. We were totally exposed to each other's unrelenting pain and each other's desperate cries.

Throughout it all, Leena and her family brought a little soul to a ward where, for the most part, there has been no soul at all. Her team mirrored my own; on either side of the hospital curtain, our two families showed what it is to love and to be loved. We may have entered each other's chapters for only a few brief pages, but we *felt* every word. I know that Leena's story will forever remain printed on my own.

Over the next few weeks, I exist in the hollow shadows she's left behind. I watch on as a constant cycle of new patients occupy the bed next door. Tonight, I stare ahead as the sheets are, once again, stripped and remade. The void where Leena once lay makes me acutely aware of the fragility of my own situation. It exposes the frightening, unpredictability of patient life.

Tonight, as the nurse switches off the lights, a doctor I've never met before emerges at the end of my bed.

'I've just been asked to give you a heads-up: we need your bed tomorrow, so it's been decided you will be discharged home in the morning.'

Discharged? Tomorrow? I stare up at him in disbelief.

'Home?'

He nods.

I turn to Mum, whose own expression reflects my panic and fear.

'But I'm still so ill.' I look up at the doctor with pleading eyes.

Acute attacks continue to explode through my body without warning, ricocheting through my limbs, sending me into extreme convulsions that last for hours. In between, I am still living in a chronic state of torture, writhing in silent agony. Still, nobody knows what this illness is or how to control my symptoms.

'How will Tilly manage at home like this?' Mum gestures to the bed, where I remain clenched in a tight ball, with a bag of frozen peas balancing on my burning head. Beneath me, cubes of ice press against my searing flank. They melt against my hot skin and seep out into my clothes, through the sheets, penetrating the mattress below. I am living in a makeshift bath. The cold is my only distraction from the unbearable pain.

'Sometimes patients are better off at home. It's a better environment.'

I think back to the day I was urgently admitted here. I was told that I *needed* to be in hospital. My condition is worse than when I arrived, but now this doctor is saying I would be better off at home.

I imagine entering my flat again and finding everything just as I left it: my favourite blanket folded across the sofa, the kettle boiling with its familiar rumble, my makeup bag sitting on the edge of the sink. Everything may look the same but in my made-up version, one fundamental thing has changed: I am discharged home with a diagnosis and treatment. I am discharged home better.

'But her attacks and symptoms still aren't under control,' Mum says. 'Tilly can't manage at home like this.'

I dream of climbing into my own bed, melting into my own pillow and wrapping myself in my own duvet, but this is a mere fantasy. It won't be cosy and gentle and calm because escaping hospital does not mean escaping this cruel illness. It will follow me like a dark shadow everywhere I go. Returning home means accepting this illness as my life. I am tormented by everything about my existence behind the hospital curtain but I also know I am exactly where I need to be. For as long as I am here in hospital, the possibility remains that one day someone could walk in and say, 'Tilly, we've found it and we're going to get you better.' Today is not that day.

The doctor shifts from foot to foot.

'Maybe you could be seen as an outpatient?' he says.

'Under who?' Mum asks.

So many different parts of my body are failing. No discipline will claim me here *in* a hospital. Out there, I'll fall even further through the gaps of a crumbling system, forgotten and hidden from view.

He pauses.

'It will be a case of comfort care.'

'*Comfort care?*' I echo back his phrase.

Mum manoeuvres onto the soaking wet mattress and wraps her arms around me.

'Palliative care,' I whisper, glancing between Mum and the doctor.

I know this doctor is saying they will make me comfortable while I wait to die. His words extinguish my final ember of hope. They snuff out that last burning wick, plummeting my world into darkness. A wispy tendril of smoke is all that remains. There is nothing comforting about hope succumbing to fear.

Mum leans into my dripping wet hair, nestling her head against mine.

'I don't understand.' My voice is shaky.

When I first arrived here, the medics seemed united in fighting this battle with me. They were all behind me, devising strategies, plotting new avenues and formulating plans. They were intent on leading me to victory. Now, after weeks stagnating in no-man's land, my comrades' fighting spirit has dwindled. The enemy is drawing in and I am being instructed to surrender. Day one, they were preparing me to live. Now, they are preparing me to die.

The doctor's bleep rings out. With that, he rushes from the blue box.

'I don't understand. I don't understand . . .' I turn to Mum, as the blue curtain flutters in his wake. 'How can they resort to "comfort care" when they haven't done all the tests?'

Mum curls up behind me and holds me in her arms. For the rest of the night I cry and I cry and I cry. I'm conscious of keeping all the other patients awake but my tears will not stop. Mum always knows what to say but tonight even she has no words. I ball my eyes out. I utter words no parent wants to hear. My present is torture and I can see no future. This can't be how this story ends.

At 3am, there's a little movement behind my curtain. A face peeps through. An elderly lady steps forward. She's wearing a hospital gown.

'I'm so sorry,' Mum whispers. 'We must be keeping you awake.'

The lady's kind eyes radiate warmth as she looks upon my bed. In front of her lies a broken mother, holding a broken daughter, two bodies intertwined among a wet mess of scrunched-up sheets and melted ice, two souls irrevocably connected by a love stronger than any pain.

'Please don't be sorry. Your tears struck me here.' The lady places her hand across her heart. 'They are angel tears.'

I have kept them locked away for so long but tonight, there are too many tears in my heart. Sometimes our tears speak what words cannot. Mine burst from me; Mum's trickle down her cheeks. I look towards the perfect stranger standing at the end of my bed. Her eyes mist over with a watery glaze. Tonight, our tears connect us as human beings.

Mum leans over my crumpled body. She looks at me with unwavering conviction. We both know that in this moment, she doesn't have a plan. All she can do is find a way to get me through.

'Tilly, you have to hold on. Hold on just a little bit longer – not for the life you are currently living but for the one that is waiting for you.'

Tonight, I am suspended somewhere between the living and the lost, tethered to the world only by a fragile thread. Yet, even now, a tiny part of me still, somehow, believes there are more chapters in this story.

I know I have to hold on.

EPILOGUE

Towards the end of that London hospital admission, I was told all the tests had been done and I could only be offered 'comfort care'. At my most desperate, I decided to share my story on Instagram and ask the world for ideas. The world answered.

I received hundreds of messages from scientists, PhD students, professors, medics, patients and families who went out of their way to share test recommendations, diagnosis suggestions and treatment options. Mum and I compiled all of their ideas into a list. We saw, firsthand, the power of social media for social good. It restored our faith in human beings.

After almost three months in hospital, I was discharged without a diagnosis. I was told to give up searching and to accept this as my life. Mum and I stood by our mantra that 'giving up is never an option'.

In the year that followed, we once again resumed our roles as medical detectives. During this time, we revisited the list from my incredible Instagram followers again and again. Mum meticulously worked her way through each and every suggestion. If it was a no, she crossed it off. If she felt it may fit, she researched further. It proved Mum's view: 'there is *always* something else'.

There was one idea we kept returning to: vascular compressions. These are a group of conditions where blood vessels become squashed, restricting blood flow to vital organs.

Mum pored over medical journals and case studies related to vascular compressions and began to notice that the name of a professor in Germany kept appearing. With no one looking into my case in the UK anymore, she proposed a new plan.

In November 2023, we boarded a plane to Germany. There, I received a diagnosis of multiple vascular compressions and went on to have three lifesaving surgeries.

While in Germany, I descended into the same metabolic crisis I had in the UK. The medics, once again, struggled to diagnose me. When it was beginning to feel hopeless, a junior doctor, who I have since taken to calling 'Dr House', overheard me sharing details of my case. This sparked an idea. While Maverick in London was restricted by systemic barriers, Dr House was given the freedom to pursue his theory. In Germany, despite me still not having a positive porphyria result, the system allowed me to trial the heme treatment. I transformed and this proved to be a vital clue that led to my final diagnosis.

Eventually, I was diagnosed, treated and cured of severe heavy metal poisoning. At last, I had an explanation for *all* my symptoms.

In Germany, I observed medical science evolving in front of my very eyes, leading to breakthroughs that have now not only saved my own life but also the lives of other patients all around the world.

I realised I was wrong: thinking and kindness are only a winning combination if they exist within a system that allows them to flourish.

What happened to me was a domino effect that required medical detective work and a holistic approach to uncover. It turned out there really was a reason for *every one* of my symptoms and they were all connected.

In Germany, the medics also identified that I'd actually been born with hypermobile Ehlers-Danlos syndrome (EDS), a condition that gives you abnormally stretchy connective tissue.

EDS makes you bendy on the outside but can make you bendy on the inside too. If a person with EDS loses a significant amount of weight, particularly at a time when things in the body are moving anyway, like during puberty, organs and veins can end up shifting and stretching into the wrong places.

Aged 14, I lost over 6kg in weight in two months because of the tuberculosis. This extreme weight loss, against the background of EDS, caused multiple vascular compressions to develop. These remained undetected for years.

My primary vascular compression was centred around my left renal vein, directly connected to my kidneys. This compression was disrupting the blood flow to my adrenal glands, causing my Addison's disease.

For years, my left renal vein compression meant my kidneys were failing to filter toxins out of my body. This resulted in a buildup of heavy metals in my tissues and blood, culminating in severe heavy metal poisoning.

Heavy metal poisoning disrupts the body's metabolic pathways and can cause a rare variant of porphyria.

You could call this a totally imperfect perfect storm.

Mine is a story about not being limited by a label. We don't say that only 'accountants' can do maths or that only 'authors' can be good at writing or that only 'historians' can understand the past, but there does often appear to be a view that only 'doctors' can understand medicine.

Aged 17, my mum was forced to leave school without any qualifications and live alone. Over the last 20 years, I've watched her go on to engage in discussions with top medical professionals on everything from multi-drug-resistant bacteria to cytochrome P450, corticosteroid-binding globulin and acute intermittent porphyria. Her relentless research and unwavering belief have shown me what can be achieved if you choose to see possibilities, rather than obstacles.

Every stage of my journey has been a battle: a battle to be believed, a battle to be diagnosed and, eventually, a battle to be treated. Throughout it all, enduring hope remained. This never just appeared on a whim; it required extreme effort, tenacity, unrelenting willpower and courage to keep that hope alive.

Over the years, whenever my path felt dark and futile, Mum, Dad, Finn and Auntie were my constant flickers of light. Just having them close by, loving me, guiding me and believing in me, allowed me to keep seeing the next step. At different stages, other people ignited our flames, allowing us to burn a little brighter. Some came in the form of revolutionary medical breakthroughs, others with a simple cup of tea. Every single one mattered. I have learned that it is the *people* who shape the patient experience.

Day one, I used so much energy trying to hide my situation, determined to be 'Tilly', not 'Tilly the patient', but over time I realised that people can't be there for you if you never let them in. The more I opened up, the more I recognised that *Be Patient* is *everyone's* story. Far from being alone, billions of people are having to navigate patient life and everyone has their own tale to tell. The reality is that we will *all* be a patient at some point in our lives. It will affect each and every one of us.

Unlike in other situations, when it all feels too much, as patients we can't just walk away. We may be prescribed medical treatment for our condition but there is no magic cure to wipe away the stories that unfold. These stay with us for life. We grow a thicker skin, in order to get through. We grow a bigger heart as well.

When life is so tough and the future uncertain, the little things end up meaning more. We savour seeing the blue sky, walking through a lush green field, sipping on a frothy coffee and laughing with friends. These small wins are fleeting reminders that moments which once seemed impossible can exist again.

Hold on.

AUTHOR'S ACKNOWLEDGEMENTS

Both being a patient and writing this book really has taken a team, and I have been so lucky to have been surrounded by some of the very best.

To Alice Saunders, your energy and enthusiasm for my writing, and for the wider impact you felt *Be Patient* could have on patient care, meant I instantly *knew* you were the agent for me!

To Nicki Kennedy, you went out of your way to support me with my writing, when I was effectively a perfect stranger. Your belief, guidance and words of encouragement compelled me to keep going.

To my editor, Mala Sanghera-Warren, it certainly hasn't been the standard editor/author relationship; we've worked together on *Be Patient* from two different countries, while I've been writing from a hospital bed. Somehow we did it and I am so proud of the book we have created!

To Sybella Stephens, Mel Four and everyone in the Octopus team, a huge thank you for believing in *Be Patient* and providing me with the platform to bring the patient voice to the forefront.

To Team Tilly:

Mum, over the years, you often said you wished you 'had a magic wand' so you could make it all go away. You didn't have a wand, but you did have a mind that never stopped thinking, a body that never stopped going and a heart that never stopped loving. You set out to save my life but along the way, you have changed and saved the lives of patients all around the world. *Be Patient* is also your life's work.

Dad, you commuted to hospitals around the UK and abroad and treated it like you were just popping down the road, while working full-time throughout. However dark it felt, you somehow managed to bring humour into every situation and always made me laugh and smile. That mattered, it really mattered.

Finn, you ensured I always knew that regardless of what happened next, we were in this *together*. 'I'm not going anywhere,' is a line you have repeated to me over the years. There have been moments when it has felt utterly hopeless but you never stopped believing that I would 'BEAT IT'.

Auntie, you have always been so special to us, but alternating with Mum, night and day, for almost three months in a hard wooden chair next to my bed, on that London hospital admission, you showed me love in its rawest form. You are like another limb to Mum and me; we love you, we trust you and we can always rely on you. Your belief has been part of my cure.

To Ogo, Sukai, Vanessa, Ava, Abebi, Rosalind, Leena, Safa and Beate for restoring my faith in human beings.

To Marguerite, for continuing to hold my tears in your heart.

To Maverick, you are a different kind of doctor and the world needs more of YOU.

To my GP, Brian, you offered me the continuity of care I was unable to get in any other area of the healthcare system.

To Professor Scholbach, Professor Sandmann, Dr Schmitz and

Dr Al-Khayat for giving hope to me and so many others, when it felt like there was no hope at all.

To Dr Hüseyin Sahinbas, Nurse Diana Sahinbas, Dr (TR) Bengisu Güvercinci- Sahinbas and most of all, Dr (TR) Ertugrul Pascal Sahinbas (aka Dr House), you didn't just save my life, you actively fought to give me a life.

To Ahmad, Andrea, Anna, Eda, Ellie, Eva, Irina, Jana L, Jana T, Julia, Karin, Kerstin H, Kerstin S, Lisa, Melanie E, Melanie S, Olga K, Olga P, Omar, Ramez, Ridwan, Schiwa, Tala, Tanja, Viktoria and Ziba, you held my hand in some of my most challenging moments.

To TB Alert, Addison's Disease Self-Help Group, Metabolic Support UK and Ehlers-Danlos Support UK, thank you for the valuable support and information you are providing for patients.

To the Parrs, know that Auntie's momentous input on this journey has not only changed my life, but impacted patient care on a global scale.

To Auntie Joan, for turning up at hospital armed with picnic hampers of tasty, nutritious treats and for lighting candles of hope for me around the world.

To Rosemary and Oliver, for bringing the best person I know into this world, and of course for Smudge, our very own therapy dog. To Oscar, Benedict, Charlotte, Archie, Haalah, Solenne, Arno, Orson and Ali – I'm excited for all the family fun with you in my new life!

To all the Devs, who have lived this journey with us from day one. You really are our family. To Guri and Rory, you shaped my childhood; your house became my second home. To Sharon and Neil, for the 'Don't Stop Me Now' moments. To Gill and Steve, for reminding me that 'the sun'll come out tomorrow'. To Simon, for always making me laugh out loud. To Chris and Sarah, for thinking of me as your daughter. To Tracy, for finding prosecco moments during tough times. To the Matthews, for all the happy family gatherings. To Mandy, for making me believe I could somehow get into Oxford University *without* going to school.

To Em, for being like a sister from the day I was born and for the all-nighters in hospital by my side. To Mel, for never ceasing to make me laugh and visualising happier times ahead. To Maddy, for being the 'pea in my pod' from our first day at playgroup and for delivering a taste of home. To Ella, for a childhood of adventures and for constantly keeping my dandelion in bloom. To Katy, for never leaving my side during that first horrific adrenal attack and for curling up on the sofa with me whenever I was too ill to go out. To Issy, for having the warmest heart and always finding ways to show how much you care. To Lottie, for a flatshare filled with laughter and love, even when things were seriously beginning to spiral. To Tess and Laura, for bringing all the gossip to the hospital wards. To Anna, for the constant supply of care packages. To Chloe, for showing from our very first day, that university friends really are friends for life. To Sophia, for thinking up the kindest gestures and organising them like a queen. To Charlotte, for *feeling* everything I have gone through and to you and Jack, for hosting wedding 'Take Two', a day I will remember forever.

To my uni & Bucks group – you are all the epitome of fun and I'm manifesting a future of holidays and parties together!

To Derek and Nina your words became a faith to 'Team Tilly'. You kept the bud of hope alive.

Finally, to my loyal @thattillyrose Instagram community, I cannot believe how you have *felt* every word of my online chapters. In our darkest moments, your beautiful messages have compelled my team and me to keep going. Your own stories have touched my heart so much that changing patient care isn't a choice anymore. This is just the beginning.

To all the incredibly brave patients I have met along the way, you are all dandelions.

ABOUT THE AUTHOR

Tilly Rose is an author and activist, championing access to higher education and patient advocacy.

After 20 years as a patient, Tilly made the decision to share her patient journey on Instagram and saw first-hand how her experiences resonated with followers. She now shares her personal story in 'chapters' on @thattillyrose, and recently launched @thatpatientcollective – a platform for other patients to share their stories and support each other along the way.

Be Patient is Tilly's first memoir and part of her wider mission to impact patient care.

@thattillyrose
@thatpatientcollective
www.thatpatientcollective.com
@thatoxfordgirl
www.thatoxfordgirl.com

This monoray book was crafted and published by
Helena Sutcliffe, Mala Sanghera-Warren, Sybella Stephens,
Monica Hope, Mel Four and Katherine Hockley.